# JUST BREATHE

# JUST BREATHE

**Andy Drooker**

Cover Design: cutting-edge-studio.com/
Editor: Amy Pattee Colvin
Breathe lyrics © Universal Music Publishing Group, Spirit Music Group, BMG Rights Management, Sony/ATV Music Publishing LLC

ISBN 9798553275525

# DEDICATION

Life happens.

In my life, I have been blessed to have had the privilege to meet and know some of the most wonderful people. I can actually say, "Knowing these people has truly changed my life."

In everyone's life, one or two people often come to mind where you can look back and say, "If it was not for...I would not be the person I am today." Well, I am honored to have known several people, and I would like to share their influences on me with those of you who are taking the time to read this dedication.

Before I share my life journey with you, let me frame-up where I was in my life when the most influential person came into my life and put me on "the right path." I was fifteen. It was the summer before my junior year of high school (or as some people like to call it, Hell School). I was living with my mom, my grandmother, and my brother. My brother was my best friend.

I had friends in high school, but I could not do a lot with them. Money was very tight growing up. My bro and I would do things together—play Atari until four in the morning, go to the comic book store, play on the computer, and so on. We shared everything growing up.

One summer evening, our grandmother introduced me to Dr. John Hutcheson, Jr. He was the Director and creator of The Center for Public and Urban Research (CPUR) at Georgia State University.

He offered me a summer job working with his staff and him on research projects. I did data entry, learned Fortran, SPSS, and mastered the skill of how to write research papers. The best part was I would earn over $3.55 an hour—great pay for the 1980s, a fortune for a junior in high school.

At the time, the school system I was in had a special program called Vocational Office Training (VOT). I went to school from 8 a.m. to 12:30 p.m. Then, I'd work at CPUR from 2 p.m. to 6 p.m. It took me an hour to get to GSU by bus every day, and the same amount of time to get home. So, I generally arrived home by seven in the evening, would eat dinner, do homework, and repeat.

During the first quarter of my junior year, I started applying to colleges. Guess which one I got into before Thanksgiving?

After I graduated high school, John offered me a full-time job. So, here I was in my first year of college, and I had a full-time campus job in a field that two years prior, I didn't even know I'd be interested in. Honestly, when I look back, I realize John gave me something so rare—direction, purpose, a life meaning, and most importantly, he gave me his time and mentored me. Without him, I do not want to think about what my life would have been like. On top of what he did for me, he took my brother under his tutelage also.

John took it upon himself to make this health journey with me. Although he is no longer with us, he will always be with me. I hope upon reading this dedication, you will get a sense of the kind of individual he was and the profound effect he had on my life.

Two other people changed my life. Bev B. and Larry G. Both were my perspective bosses/mentors at Turner Broadcasting. I will go into greater detail about these extraordinary individuals who, like John H., took a chance on me. They let me grow as an individual and a leader within their organization. But, most importantly, they treated me with respect and as their equal. Words cannot express my appreciation, gratitude, and respect I have for them to this day. Just know, the relationship I had with them went beyond friendship and was more in-line with family.

# CONTENTS

# OPENING THOUGHTS

**Cope**
Verb (used without object)
To face and deal with responsibilities, problems, or difficulties, especially successfully or in a calm or adequate manner.
–dictionary.com

**Cope**
Verb (intransitive verb)
1a: to deal with and attempt to overcome problems or difficulties.
1b: to maintain a contest or combat usually on even terms or with success.
–Merriam-Webster

*Sounds simple enough, right?*

**Hope**
Verb (intransitive verb)
To cherish a desire with anticipation: to want something to happen or be true.
–Merriam-Webster

> It was the best of times; it was the worst of times.
> –Charles Dickens

The above quote sums up my life perfectly. I have lived a wonderfully rich, rewarding life. I have had the opportunity to be part of so many wonderful things that I could fill another book—from a career launching networks for Ted Turner around the world, to the best job any man could hope to get, being a father.

I am a father to a gorgeous, insightful, creative daughter. Who, I hope, will have her own view of the world someday. But along that journey, she will hopefully give her dad some gray hair, not a lot, while keeping him young.

For most of my life, unknown to me, I have lived with and battled with cystic fibrosis (CF). As you continue reading, I'll walk you on the journey I took to get to this very point; you will understand how for forty-nine years, I fought with it and did not even know it. For every breath I take—thanks, Sting—it affects my body. Sleeping with this unknown enemy takes its toll.

The battle rages on several fronts. First is the psychological front. That front is composed of a three-pronged assault on me, my mind, and my heart.

What weapons do I utilize in my arsenal? I cannot be like Captain Kirk—you will see a lot of Star Trek metaphors, more on that later—and fire phasers, thus destroying the enemy. No, my weapons are inside me—attitude, emotional strength, and determination.

Falling into a mind-field of self-pity and self-doubt is sometimes easy. When those two attack slowly, the defenses are not always strong enough, and the darkness creeps in. When that occurs, hoping and coping are just words with no meaning, no power, not a defense. Nothing has any meaning.

My sighs of desperation, frustration, and shaky self-worth instigated a fire in my mind to share the importance of my story. This book is not so much a memoir as it is a legacy for my daughter. It is a book about surviving and growing. Rising above, fear, anger, self-pity, doubt, and let's not forget the anger caused by the question anyone would ask, "Why the fuck me?"

So, the book is not about illness, but about the quest for emotional and physical health. If you are looking for the answer, there is only an answer—coping, taking the journey of a personal quest for answers and peace. This book describes my path. Remember, living life is not about the destination; it is about the journey. If you have ten ways to cross town, all will help you arrive at your destination, but the one you choose to follow is up to you.

This story is my journey. I sincerely hope you enjoy the ride with me. We will make stops, but they all are necessary because they got me to where I am today and will most likely be tomorrow.

One last note, learning to cope is the toughest part of any education. School is always in session. It is never over. New situations and challenges arise daily, which requires never-ending adjustments. Learning to live with adversity is instinctive. If something is instinctive, an individual will naturally or automatically, inherently self-learn and adapt to the situation. That is what life is. Yes, it sucks! But, if it was really that bad, would I want to share it with you?

That is the question, or did I already give my answer?

And the adventure continues...

# PREFACE—WHY WRITE A BOOK?

> Do not go where the path may lead, go instead where there is no path and leave a trail.
> –Ralph Waldo Emerson

At birth in December 1965, I was not diagnosed with any life-threatening illness. It was not until I was three years of age that I was diagnosed with asthma. Asthma is a condition in which your airways narrow, swell, and produce extra mucus. This makes breathing difficult and may trigger coughing, wheezing, and shortness of breath. For some people, asthma is a minor nuisance. However, for me, it caused visits to the hospital many, many times.

The biggest issue I faced with asthma was getting pneumonia. Pneumonia is an infection that inflames the air sacs in one or both lungs. The air sacs may fill with fluid or pus—purulent material—causing cough with phlegm or pus, fever, chills, and difficulty breathing. A variety of organisms, including bacteria, viruses, and fungi, can cause pneumonia.

I was in the hospital yearly. But my parents and brother always by my side; everyone figured, hey it is just asthma.

Fast forward to my forty-ninth year on earth, when I am working for a large logistics company—

after a long and successful career in media working for some of the most wonderful people I have met on my life's journey.

While working for this logistics company, I traveled a lot and enjoyed my job. However, I noticed that I began to have above-average difficulty breathing, and I was tiring quickly. Just taking a shower caused shortness of breath. Walking from the corporate parking lot to my office was exhausting. Something was wrong, but what!?

Well, since you already know this book is about my journey with CF, you can guess what came next—doctor visits and trips to various specialists. At the end of that long road, I was finally diagnosed with CF. Many tests and events occurred in the time from the start of the journey to a discovery of the true diagnosis; I will discuss all of this, and more, later.

Cystic fibrosis is a serious genetic disorder with reduced life expectancy. Mutations cause disorder in the cystic fibrosis transmembrane conductance regulator (CFTR) gene, which regulates the production of mucus, sweat, and digestive enzymes. For an individual to have CF, both his or her parents have to be carriers of this mutated CFTR gene.

Discovered and named in the 1930s, the name cystic fibrosis refers to the characteristic scarring (fibrosis) and cyst formation within the pancreas. It is estimated that more than 70,000 people worldwide are living with CF, but the incidence of the disease varies across the world. The United States is among one of the countries with the highest incidence of CF, with about 30,000 people currently living with the disease. Approximately 1,000 new cases of CF are diagnosed each year in the United States, with more than seventy-five percent being diagnosed by the age of two. CF is a childhood disease.

Life expectancy for patients with CF has greatly increased in the past few years. The median age of survival for a person with CF is around forty-seven years. However, patients like myself are living well into their fifties and, if they are lucky, into their sixties. Please note, these statistics do not take into account patients who have had lung transplants. I am still utilizing my original lungs.

A quick note about lung transplants—transplanted lungs, on average, give a CF patient five years of use. The lungs are the only organ to be constantly exposed to the outside air. Therefore, a patient who has transplanted lungs must take various medications daily to avoid infection, sepsis, organ rejection, and just daily irritants in the air. A common cold can cause a CF patient to drown in their mucus. There is no cure for CF.

As my time in this world was now perpetually in doubt, I came to realize that CF has had a dramatic effect on my life. As I approach and pass the age which my mother left this world, I look back and marvel at how I have cheated death for so long. Keep in mind this is the first book written by anyone with CF who had no idea they had CF growing up. I seemed fine, until one day, my breathing became excessively labored. Then, everything changed.

For people who know the surface of me, they see a divorced man—**more about that later**—trying to get back into the workforce, and a father of a beautiful daughter, who is my life and my light.

As a father, I was forced to fight a legal battle to illustrate that having CF does not make one an incapable parent—**more on this later**—as my ex-wife wanted to convince the courts. This potential court case clearly illustrated that CF is not well known or understood and cannot be easily seen or even properly imagined by most people. Cystic fibrosis seems to be one of those diseases where some feel that if it can't be seen, it doesn't exist—ignorance is a form of **prejudice**. All the damage from the illness is on the inside, both physically and mentally.

Historically, I tended to suppress all my emotions and feelings about my condition. I have been guarded about disclosing it to strangers. I never wanted to be viewed as a sick person or be defined by my condition. Lastly, I never wanted anyone to feel sorry for or pity me—what example would that set for my daughter? However, after years of secrecy and guardedness, I'm left with a significant amount of unresolved sadness and emotion.

But, hey, I am defying the odds. I lived past the average! Surviving CF has been a big achievement in my life; however, my biggest success and legacy in this life will always be my daughter and the memories I will leave behind. Hence, my life and those that have been with me is something I want to share with the world. How and what did I do all those years not knowing I had CF, that kept me alive? Consider all the medications I was taking for asthma, did they help or hurt?

An old saying suggests, "What cannot be cured, needs to be endured." As I reflected on my life journey, I realized I had some extraordinary stories to share. The things I have seen, the people who made me into the person typing these words for you. I want the world to know that it is these people, places, and experiences that define oneself, not CF or any illness or handicap. I hope by reading this story of my life, it will give you hope and perseverance and optimism about yours. So, onto my life story.

It began on a dark and stormy night...

# Breathe
### Alexi Murdoch

In the quiet of the shadow
In the corner of a room
Darkness moves upon you
Like a cloud across the moon
You're a-wearing all the silence
Of a constant that will turn
Like the windmill left deserted
Or the sun forever burn
So don't forget to breathe
Don't forget to breathe
Your whole life is here
No eleventh-hour reprieve
So don't forget to breathe
Keep your head above water
But don't forget to breathe
And all the suffering that you've witnessed
And the handprints on the wall
They remind you how it's endless
How endlessly you fall
And the answer that you're seeking
For the question that you found
Drives you further to confusion
As you lose your sense of ground
So don't forget to breathe
Don't forget to breathe
Your whole life is here
No eleventh-hour reprieve
So don't forget to breathe

Keep your head above water
But don't forget to breathe
Breathe
Don't forget to breathe
Don't forget to breathe
You know you are here
But you find you want to leave
So don't forget to breathe
Just breathe
Just breathe
Just breathe
Just breathe
Just breathe

# 1: THE END/THE BEGINNING

Do the difficult things while they are easy and
the great things while they are small. A
journey of a thousand miles must begin with a
simple step.
–Lao Tzu

The journey begins.

"You have six months to live unless you get a lung transplant!" My journey started the moment I heard that statement.

At the time, I worked at a global logistics company. Traveling and working on large IT projects that kept me out of town for weeks. As I traveled, I noticed that I was tired and out-of-breath more frequently. For my whole life, I knew I had asthma. So, I figured I'd just use my rescue inhaler to keep me going. It was all good, except I was going through the inhalers quicker then I could legally refill them at the pharmacy.

It was time for me to call my asthma doctor, Dr. Degryse. Now, normally when I went to Dr. Degryse, I "assumed the position" and received a steroid shot—these are not the steroids that Mark McGwire would take; no, these open up my breathing airways. The shot did two things. One, it improved my breathing. Two, I got a case of the munches and visited Waffle House to gain some weight—which for me was not a bad thing.

I arrived at the doctor's office, and they checked for normal vitals. But, this time, nothing was normal. I sat on the exam table and zoned-out. In came the doctor, who said something I didn't process. Did my doctor just tell me I have six months to live?

"What, wait?! Are you sure you are in the right room?" I commented, then continued, "I just came in for a shot for my breathing. You know, the normal steroid shot that helps me breathe and gives me the munchies!" I said, laughing—I'm good at using humor as a defense mechanism. I glanced at my lovely doctor, who always had a smile on her face; she was not smiling. She was staunch, rigid, and had a serious look on her face.

"Your oxygen saturation reading for your blood is eighty-one percent. That is very low. Normally someone with that reading should be in the hospital. There is no way I can let you go back to work. If you go back to work, it will just speed up the process." She stated.

I asked, "What process?"

Her response came, with no pause or hesitation, "Dying."

At that point, I felt the blood and color drain from my face. I heard my heartbeat in my head.

She continued, "Andy, listen to me, if your company has a short-term disability program, you need to get that paperwork for me to complete. You need to go on disability so we can find out what is wrong with you while we have time. I will complete all the paperwork needed."

"Okay, I will do that, but what is my diagnosis? What do I have that could have caused such a decrease in my body's ability to process oxygen? Why do I need a lung transplant? I feel fine. Just tired and out of breath. If you were traveling and working the hours I have been, I am sure you would be tired also. That's why I came in for my regular shot." I stated, with a touch of panic in my voice.

My doctor was silent for a moment, then continued, "Mr. Drooker..." when she addressed me in this manner, I knew she was trying to let me know to take this seriously. When someone calls you "Mr.," it's like hearing your parents call you by your first and middle name, you are in trouble!

She continued, "I am going to take x-rays, some blood, and do a pulmonary function test (PFT). The PFT will tell us what your lung capacity is. The x-ray will tell us if it is something simple like a collapsed lung, and the blood-work will tell us if you have an infection."

In my head, I thought, "...something simple like a collapsed lung. Is she fucking serious!? I would be in excruciating pain. Never-mind, lightheaded, dizzy, and my chest would feel like a huge weight is pushing against it."

"Great, let's get started," I said, encouraged. I thought perhaps the oxygen sensor was faulty. I know technology. I know equipment makes or gives bad readings all the time, especially if the batteries have not been changed. "Yeah, that's got it be it, old batteries," I thought to myself. There goes that defense mechanism again.

Hours passed. I finished a graphic novel while waiting. Finally, the doctor entered the little exam room, closed the door slowly, and started talking.

"We know something is going on in your lungs. But according to the x-rays, everything looks normal. Your white blood cell count is slightly elevated. That could mean you are fighting something, but what it is, remains to be discovered. In the meantime, I am prescribing oxygen for you as well as an antibiotic. The $O_2$ will help you breathe easier and might help with the level of exhaustion you are feeling.

You need to make an appointment with the lung-transplant team at Emory Healthcare. This will start the long process of getting evaluated and put on the list for new lungs. Then, make an appointment with an infectious disease physician. Before you can be placed on the transplant list, we need to diagnose you. Unfortunately, you have something that I cannot diagnose."

"Wait, let me understand this. You have no idea what I have, but you do know that I need a new set of lungs to live past six months? So, the $O_2$ and the pills are for what?" she could hear the frustration in my voice.

"The $O_2$ and pills are to keep you alive. If you did not come in here today, more than likely, you would have eventually passed-out or fainted, and at that point, the road to recovery would have been a dead-end." She stated.

"Pardon the pun, right?" I quipped back.

She smiled and said, "It is not going to be easy, but your life today is now totally different than it was yesterday."

What a difference a day makes. How right she was. Little did I know that over the next several months, I would embark on a life-changing journey but not with my wife, with my mentor. I was angry, then scared. Why was this happening now? My wife, at the time, was six months from having our first child. I was the main breadwinner. What were we, soon to be I, going to do?

# 2: DAD

I've always had a particular affinity for father-
son dramas.
–Robert Picardo

"Try it on. Let's see how you look," became a phrase I often heard from my father. My first suit. My first men's watch, my school uniform, when I attended Fessenden School in Massachusetts, my first razor to shave, which to this day I hate doing. In each instance, his face always had the same expression—a beaming sense of pride.

Some of my favorite memories as a child and teenager were days when my dad took my brother and me to Pine Brook Country Club. Although Pine Brook was a Country Club, we never saw it in that light.

We would swim, play tennis, or try to, and fish in a lake that was on the 13th hole! Yep, our dad would take us out in a golf-cart, with all our fishing gear, and we'd fish while people are playing golf around us. What we caught we often threw back, but every now-and-then we would keep a fish, freshwater Bass, bring it into the kitchen of the Grill Room, and our dad or a family friend would eat it! But the most fun was playing golf with our dad—which generally entailed driving the carts at high speeds.

Although our parents divorced, my brother and I always had our father in our lives. While not physically in our home, he was involved to what extent he could be.

Nowadays, we live in a fatherless generation. Fifty-seven point six percent of African-American children, thirty-one point two percent of Hispanic children, and twenty point seven percent of white children live without their biological father. Millions more have dads who are physically present but emotionally absent. So when people hear the word "Father" or read these statistics, they shudder or remember the vacant spot where their dad should have been.

But a father is not one who simply has paternal claims to you. Being a father means so much more than a man who lives in the same house as his children.

In comic books, one of the most well-known and respected storylines of a father is Jonathan Kent—Superman's adopted earth father. Clark Kent is nowhere near close to a biological son and, with his powers alone, presents the possibility of inviting unwanted problems into the Kent household. Yet, Jonathan raises him as his own flesh and blood.

Seeing such world-changing potential in his son, Jonathan Kent sacrifices his comfort to hide Clark until he's ready. When Clark stumbles, Jonathan's the anchor to return him to his path of greatness. He never gives up on Clark and always holds the belief his adopted son could be the hope people need. And Clark does just that. He becomes a beacon of hope to a dying world.

There was a man in my life besides my father, who formed me into the person I am today. A man who showed me what it was like to honor, love, romance, and respect a woman. A man who emulated courage and humility. A man who picked me up when I fell. A man who held fast to the belief I can be so much more. That man was discussed in the dedication.

Growing up with two geographic homes was normal for my brother and me. During the school year, we would be with our mom in Florida and later in Georgia. During the summer months and various winter breaks, we would be with our father in Boston. Sometimes on special holidays, like Thanksgiving, our father would come to us. I think that is why, to this day, Thanksgiving holds a special meaning in my heart.

My father grew up in a manicured home with my grandparents. My grandmother was stereotypical of her era. My grandfather, a veteran of World War II, started his own business to contribute to the ever-growing need for upholstery for automobiles.

My grandparents had two children, my father and his sister, whom I never met. From what I was told, she was very intelligent and loving but lived in a world by herself. Tragedy struck my father at a young age when his older sister committed suicide. He never talked about her or what happened. One has to remember that time, in the 1950s and 1960s, family issues were kept very private. No one would ask; oddities would simply go undiscussed.

My father always had a picture of her somewhere in his home. I am not sure if he had it to remind himself of her or remind himself that he, too, was alone and ultimately responsible for his parents. I suppose it does not matter in the end. He was there for his parents and his sons.

# 3: MOM

Most mothers are instinctive philosophers.
-Harriet Beecher Stowe

As a child of a divorced home, my brother and I were primarily raised by our mother, who had MS.

I witnessed first-hand in my mother the qualities I would, for the rest of my life, associate with heroism. She had what seemed to me, in retrospect, a near-limitless capacity for kindness. She was deeply empathic and compassionate. She taught us to never tease someone for something they could not change about themselves.

She was devoted to family, friends even when they did not deserve it, and she had a seemingly bottomless well of love and willingness to sacrifice, at great cost to her, to ensure that we had a childhood of innocence and joy. She gave until she had nothing left and then gave some more, largely to ensure that we could pursue our dreams and live in hope, even when she could not.

# 4: I ARRIVED

The more complex the mind, the greater need
for the simplicity of play.
–J.T. Kirk

It was a dark and stormy winter night in the year is 1965. The month was December. The time was three in the morning. The weather was twenty-seven degrees with light snow. This was the day I arrived in this world.

What else was happening on the day of my birth? The world had a state funeral for Winston Churchill, the United States used chemical weapons in Vietnam, and Lyndon Johnson signed the voting rights act. On the entertainment front, the Sound of Music was released, and the second Star Trek pilot went into production.

Our first home was a 1960s style ranch house in Weston, Massachusetts. The main floor had the basics: a wood-paneled den-TV room, a guest room, which became my brother's room two years later, a guest bathroom, a master bedroom with a connected bathroom, my room, a living-dining room, and a kitchen with a connected playroom.

My memories of that first home are very cloudy. I see pictures of my brother and me when we were young in that home. How I wish I could go back and tell my younger self what was coming.

The memory that stands out the most about my early childhood in that home was the spooky basement. However, even if it was spooky, the basement had trains. Our father loved model trains. Over half the basement was allocated to a huge table that had old-style Tyco trains on it—tunnels, street signs, functional street lights. Dad had a deep commitment to the detailed and complex art of play. Yep, our Dad loved to build anything.

Maybe that is where my brother and I get our knack for wanting to take things apart and figure out how they work, and I'm sure this is why Ikea furniture does not bother us!

# 5: SEVENTH GRADE–FIRST REMEMBERED HOSPITAL STAY

What a superior man seeks is in himself; what the small man seeks is in others.
–Confucius

As I look back at the years spent in school leading up to the big day of high school graduation, it amazes me that I made it. Seriously! These school years offer many vivid memories, not all of them pleasant.

My first vivid memory of going into the hospital for my breathing issues happened when I was in middle school. The cycle, starting in the sixth grade, would go something like this: get sick, be diagnosed with pneumonia, and get admitted to the hospital. Then the treatment would look something like this: IVs, oxygen tents, breathing treatments, and a minimum of a week's stay.

Suffice to say, I had a lot of alone time. So, what does a seventh-grader do to keep busy in the hospital? At that time, hospital rooms didn't have TVs. If a patient wanted a TV, they had to pay a daily fee. To reiterate, we had no money; an extra $10.00 a day was a lot of money.

What kept me going? Will power and listening to my favorite TV show! I know what you are thinking, how does a seventh-grader in the '70s have the ability to listen to a favorite TV show on-demand? Video on demand was not invented yet; neither were audiobooks. So, how was I able to do this, years before it became common?

In school, I had a very noticeable stuttering handicap, and at that time, our single mom, who, as I mentioned, had MS and no steady income. She could not afford to send me to a speech pathologist or special school to overcome my stuttering. My mom spoke with several specialists on the phone; they told her my issue came from thinking so fast I'd skip over my words, which in turn caused my stuttering.

Also, being able to speak complex strings of words and enunciate correctly was another factor. I vividly remember my mom sitting me down, almost on the verge of tears, telling me that she did not have the money to send me to school to receive the help I need for my stuttering. She then wiped her face and told me, "You can help yourself."

Then she asked me in a very soft and caring voice, "What is your favorite TV show?" A question to which she already knew the answer.

"Star Trek, you know that!"

She continued, "This is what I want you to do. Take your tape recorder into the den when you are getting ready to watch your show, then record the show as you watch it. You can fit two episodes on one cassette tape. After the show, go into your room, put in an audio earplug, and listen to the actors speak their lines. Notice how they speak the lines, how they pronounce the words, and how they pause. I want you to memorize the dialog. Then say it back, out loud, to yourself."

I did that for my favorite episodes. They were a mixture of action, humor, and morality. Star Trek fans reading this can probably guess what episodes I am talking about. In any case, I recorded about ten episodes on five cassette tapes. And I listened.

Back in the hospital, my mom brought my Radio Shack cassette recorder/player to my room. All she said to me was, "I brought you some friends to study with!" While alone, in my sterile hospital room, under an oxygen tent, I listened and spoke out loud. I fell asleep listening to those episodes or reading my favorite comic book—Green Lantern, hence the power of will—and now and then, my mom would record a message for me. She could not come up to the hospital and see me that much due to her MS, but she was there with me, along with my fictional friends—yes, I know they're from a TV show— helping me get well in the real world.

By the time I reached high school, my stuttering was getting better, but it was still with me. However, on a brighter note, because of the work I did regarding speaking and memorizing lines, I had a wonderful ability to present reports in front of my classmates in the majority of classes. Sure, I still slipped up now and then, especially when my eye caught the eye of certain girls that all high school boys have crushes on!

As time and technology progressed, videotapes emerged, but I still kept up with my recordings. I moved on to movies. This treatment protocol continued into my college years and eventually to this day. Through using my interests as a strength to conquer perceived weakness, I overcame one of mine.

I have spoken in front of large crowds, and I have pitched ideas to my bosses. Every time I go into a situation that requires me to think fast, speak fast and get to the point, I always remember the words from Captain Kirk I heard over and over again, "Risk. Risk is our business..." and his monologue continues for two minutes. It energizes me to get excited about what I am doing, pitching, and more importantly, how I communicate it.

The take away from this aspect of my life is, there is always another way, even if you don't see that it is in front of you at the moment. But don't despair, if a seventh-grader, whose mom thought out of the box, can use listening to Star Trek to overcome stuttering and become a public speaker as part of his career, you, too, can overcome your challenges.

On a side note, looking back, Mom was ahead of her time. Yes, she used repetition and recordings to learn. But look at today's world, and you see audiobooks, Rosetta Stone to learn languages, VOD, and so on. If I only knew Ted Turner when I was in the seventh-grade!

And the adventure continues...

# 6: HELL SCHOOL–PEACHTREE–COLLAPSED LUNG

Did you know the inventor of the flush toilet
was named Thomas Crapper?
–Dana Scully

The time, 1984. The place Peachtree High School. It was late May when seniors get lazy. Only two more weeks of the school year remained for seniors. The first week was for finals; the weekend was senior prom; then, the last week of school was about preparing to go to college.

Needless to say, I was stressed out about finals. Why do teachers always schedule their finals on the same day as each other? Even in college, what is the deal with that?

In any case, my first final of the week was honors English. It was a comprehensive exam of all the works of Shakespeare we covered in class. I knew most of them and the themes. The material did not frighten me; it was the format of the answers that did—all essays. Spelling and punctuation counted. Like in this book! In any case, I completed the exam, turned in my blue-book, and sat quietly, waiting for the bell for the next period. The next exam was calculus. Oh, happy, happy, joy, joy!

Suddenly, out of nowhere, my chest started to get tight. I thought I was about to have an asthma attack due to the stress, but this felt different. I felt a sharp pain in my chest; every breath was labored as I tried to take in air. Then, I lost my sight! Everything turned white. My eyes were open, but I could not see anything but whiteness. My skin felt cold and clammy. I could hear people around me talking.

As soon as I put my head down on my desk, the bell rang for the next period. I heard people getting up and leaving. I had one slight problem; I couldn't see. How was I going to get from my English classroom, on one side of the school, to my next classroom completely on the other side of school without being able to see? Never mind, what the fuck is going on with me?

I got up from my chair and walked straight toward the door. I felt the door frame on my right side. The hair on my arms stood up. My sense of touch was elevated. I continued to walk straight until I hit the wall of lockers opposite the classroom I just left. "Okay, I now have a guide," I said to myself. If I continue to follow this wall, I should be able to make it to my next classroom in time.

As I started slowly walking, some of my vision returned. My head began to hurt due to the sudden influx of light. By the time I made it to my next class, I found my seat and put my head down. However, my chest hurt. Every breath I took was labored. If I took in a deep breath, the pain was at least an eight on a one to ten scale. I could not focus on anything but breathing. I know that sounds bizarre. Breathing is an autonomic function of the body, yet I needed to concentrate on ensuring I didn't breathe in too deeply, or the pain would crash over me.

I asked the teacher if I could be excused. I needed to see my Calculus Coach, Coach Redford. To this day, I have him to thank for my early achievements in mathematics and the ability to visualize a solution in my head and work backward from there. He was an inspiration to me and a caring teacher, and he had a wonderful sense of humor and sarcasm. I hope those of you reading this had at least one Coach Redford in your educational years. All it takes is one to make the hellish experience of high school bearable!

I made my way to the teacher's lounge, where Coach always drank his coffee in the morning. As I approached him, he said in his deep raspy voice, "Son, what are you doing here? Shouldn't you be getting ready for your calculus exam?"

"Coach, I am not feeling so well. What should I do?" It was the first time I'd ever said anything like that to him.

He calmly said, "And, you look like shit too! I want you to go to your car and drive home. Don't worry about checking out of school; I'll handle that for you. As far as your final goes, I will talk to Ms. Williams and get you exempt. We both know you were going to ace that test anyway. You have an A-average. She should have exempted you, to begin with. She is just annoyed that you came to me for advice. Now go, before my coffee high wears off."

I left the lounge and walked straight for my beautiful first car. It was an olive green 1968 Chevy Bel Air. It had a bench front seat, huge back seat—wink, wink—and a trunk in which you could fit four fully inflated spare tires. It might not have looked like much, but it was mine. Every time I stepped on the gas, the speedometer would go up; the gas gage would go down!

I made it home. I walked in the door and went straight to my mom's room. I told her the pain I was in. At this point, my breathing was getting shallow. The pain increased, and my ability to focus on breathing became labored. I had to concentrate.

Mom called my doctor, and he told her to take me to the hospital emergency room...now! Good thing my grandmother Nana was home as I couldn't drive myself, and because of the MS, Mom couldn't drive either. I got in my grandmother's car and passed out! She yelled at me, but all I wanted to do was close my eyes. So tired I was, so very, very tired. Blackness.

I woke up inside a hospital room. My grandmother was on the right side of the bed, looking down at me. My entire body was in a slanted position on the bed with my head below my feet. Grandmother was talking to someone outside my field of vision. I heard the other person say, "That will not work, nurse!" More blackness. No dreaming.

I woke up again. My body was still in the diagonal position on the bed, except I was waking up more. My chest was in pain. The pain rating was a ten! I looked down at my chest and saw a tube the size of a garden hose sticking out of my chest on the right side. It was a clear tube filled with blood which was connected to a vacuum bottle on the floor; gravity and the vacuum bottle combined to suck the blood out of me.

I freaked out! I thought to myself, what would Captain Kirk say to Dr. McCoy if he woke up with a fucking garden hose coming out of his chest? So, I said exactly that, "Excuse me, but can you please tell me why I have a fucking garden hose in my chest?

Oh, and while we are on the subject, what the fuck is wrong with me, where am I, and who are you?" I then continued, "Sorry, Nana, how would you feel if you woke up like this?"

Her response, classic, "Depends on who I woke up next to!"

"Nana, stop, I am sick enough! I do not need any images in my mind right now." I snapped back.

The doctor introduced himself, "I am Dr. Turk, the on-call pulmonologist. You are a very lucky young man."

"That's funny; I don't feel so lucky being in a hospital bed with a garden hose in my chest sucking the blood out of me." I quipped back.

"You had a pneumothorax." He stated calmly.

"A what? A what? What's a pneumothorax? Is it fixable?" I said, with a slight sense of humor in my voice—defense mechanism rises again.

He continued, "A pneumothorax is a technical term for a collapsed lung. It occurs when air leaks into the space between your lung and the chest wall. This air pushes on the outside of your lung and makes it collapse. By the time we got you into the room to put the, as you call it, garden hose in you, your right lung was collapsed about eighty-five percent. Your body was functioning mainly on your left lung. The blood you see in the tube is the liquid that filled the space between your lung and chest wall. Think of it as explosive decompression in your body. Do you have any questions?"

"Yes," I said calmly. "First, is it fixable? Second, it sounds like, in plain English, I was lucky to get here so quickly."

"Andy, first, yes, it is fixable. But it will take time to get all the liquid out of your lung cavity. In basic terms, once that occurs, we can start the process to re-inflate the lung. Now, the answer to your second question is, yes, you were lucky. If your lung fully deflated and liquid-filled your lung cavity, technically, you could have drowned." The doctor paused and asked, "Anything else?"

I replied, "Well, not to sound ungrateful, but what is the estimated time that I will be here? It is my senior year. I graduate in two weeks, and senior prom is this weekend and—"

He interrupted me, "I am going to push the pause button on you right there. We need to find the cause and get you back to some level of normal, so this does not happen again. We are sure it is related to your asthma. You will be here for at least a week. So, I hate to deliver bad news, but you are going to miss your senior prom." He stated in a very methodical and monotone voice.

"As a doctor, you sure do know how to deliver bad news. Have you heard of the TV show Star Trek? I only ask because you delivered that news with no emotion. Can I just call you Dr. Spock? It would make remembering names so much easier." I said with a smile.

He responded, "You are a very logical patient. I can already tell that you are going to be an interesting but rewarding case. See you tomorrow, get some sleep. Dr. Spock out!"

The next day came. Several friends from high school came up to see me. I remember all of them, and to this day, we're all still friends; however, I have no memory of what we talked about. Though if I were a betting person, I would have to say we discussed the upcoming opening of Star Trek III.

On the third day of my hospital stay, I had many visitors, including Mom, Nana, and Bro, who had just seen the latest Indiana Jones film. He told me I wouldn't like it as much as the first one. He made me feel better already! The next visitor was my boss at CPUR, John. He came up to see how I was feeling, to let me know my work is piling up in my cube, and to tell me my job was waiting for me when I got out of the hospital. It was a good day.

During the rest of my hospital stay, I had tests, x-rays, and more blood taken than I thought I had in my body! But, after a week, my lung was re-inflated. The cause of my pneumothorax was a pulmonary bleb, which was explained to me as essentially a pimple on the upper lobe of the lung. When the bleb popped, like a pimple, it essentially caused explosive decompression in the chest cavity. This, in turn, caused the lung to collapse.

In hindsight, what was interesting about this incident was at no time did anyone question the amount of liquid in my lungs. No one doubted that it was anything but a byproduct of asthma. My lung-health journey continued past this incident into my college and professional years. Little did I know that this event was a signpost that the entire medical staff on my case ignored or missed. It was discovered and identified thirty years later as a product of CF.

Speaking of college and professional years, they were quickly approaching as my tenure at CPUR and GSU became full time in the fall.

And the adventure continues...

# 7: CROSSROADS

When the solution is simple, God is answering.
-Albert Einstein

The year is 1989. I had been at the Center for Public and Urban Research (CPUR) for eight years. Things were going well. Then I heard the news that John Hutcheson was retiring from the University. My mentor, my friend, my second father, was leaving. Many different feelings and thoughts washed over me. Panic. Abandonment. Happiness for John. I could continue, but why bother; I contemplated leaving. I could not imagine working for someone else.

John left, and the Research Center fell under the purview of another university professor who had zero practical research methods training and never managed a group as large as CPUR. These were all signs to me. It was time to move on.

Since I'd worked in the public sector for so many years, I applied for several federal jobs. The Center had many clients in the Federal government; thus, I knew how their application process operated at that time. Remember, this is before the Internet, e-mail, and so forth. All applications had to be typed and mailed to the central employment office for the Federal Government in Washington, DC.

Eventually, all the manual work of submitting multiple applications paid off. I received a call from the Environmental Protection Agency (EPA) to begin the interview process. They were looking for a senior network and database administrator. The position was a GS-12, which at the time was a fairly high government position classification. In 1989 dollars, that was $28,000 per year. Wow!

Several weeks had passed while decisions were made, during which time I still applied for other positions. Finally, the EPA called, spoke to me on the phone, and decided to fly me to DC for a face-to-face interview, common in the technological dark ages of the 1980s.

The offices were across the street from the Pentagon. I was very excited. The interviewers explained before they could move any further, that the FBI needed to do a background check on me. I provided a long list of names for references and other required information. It was at this time I was informed that this position required Top Secret clearance. This meant in addition to speaking with my provided references, the FBI could interview anyone in my life, including but not limited to, my neighbors, family, friends, school professors, and whoever they deemed relevant. It was quite interesting when one of my professors pulled me aside and asked me, "What kind of trouble are you in? The FBI came to my home last night and asked me about you."

I replied, "No trouble, I just applied for a job that requires Top Secret clearance."

He continued, "It must be very secret because they asked questions for about forty-five minutes."

A month passed. I received a nondescript envelope from the federal government in the mail. I still have it to this day—no, I am not a hoarder, just a collector. The envelope's contents congratulated me on being awarded the position and notified me of my start date. Things seemed to be moving in the right direction.

Upon receiving this news, I called my mother and told her that I would be moving to DC. She was very excited for me, and asked all the motherly questions, "Are you sure this is what you want? It is so far from home!"

"Yes, this is a great opportunity for me." A few weeks later, I made my first trip to DC to look at places to live. I found a wonderfully small one-bedroom apartment in Alexandria, VA, for $650 a month. That was in my high range, but it was in a great area, near a train station and close to work.

As my odyssey to DC occurred, my mother and grandmother, with whom my brother lived, decided to move back to Florida. My grandmother was my mother's caretaker; my mom's MS was not getting better. So my grandmother, who hated the cold, decided to move to Florida, where it is warmer.

Unfortunately, this move presented a problem. My brother was in college and living with my mom and grandmother. Once they moved to Florida, he would have to either get an apartment or live on campus. Honestly, neither was an option. My brother worked hard at school and had a part-time job that paid for gas, insurance, and school supplies. Anything else was a luxury.

At this point, Mom asked me to stay in Atlanta and share an apartment with my brother; in essence, become his roommate. She would feel better knowing that we are watching over each other. I told her I would if I could get a job in Atlanta. The deck was stacked in her favor.

My brother, at the time, was working at Turner Broadcasting. His part-time job was printing out the daily programming logs for TBS/TNT master-control. It does not sound like a lot of work, but it was, given the era and the state of technology at Turner. My brother went to his boss and asked if there was a full-time technology position for me!

Guess what? His boss's boss was creating a position for the traffic group. In those days, there was no IT department. Each business unit was responsible for its own information technology (IT) needs. Traffic was part of ad sales, which was one of the many important divisions of the company at the time; it generated the revenue. No revenue, no jobs. Simple mathematics.

I must admit, I was skeptical at first. I knew nothing about the media. However, I loved the media. All through high school and college, I'd heard about Ted Turner. I respected the man for what he accomplished, starting with nothing more than a billboard company. He had a vision, which, in my opinion, still stands today. Ted always said, "Content is king; distribution is queen." In any case, I had an interview scheduled with Carol Gordon, the SVP of traffic.

I walked into the interview in a suit, with my resume, and a bit of knowledge in my head—I'd researched what I could about Turner and its humble beginnings. Carol was very direct. She asked questions regarding my technical skills, my thoughts about being a department of one, and my feelings about jumping right in to solve problems that Ted wanted to be solved yesterday.

I was equally direct with my answers, which she appreciated. She then proceeded to tell me that since this position was not budgeted at the beginning of the year, I would have to meet with Mr. Turner—he had to approve all hires whose position was not planned for at the beginning of the fiscal year.

My heart skipped a beat. I started to break-out in a cold sweat. Carol walked me down to Mr. Turner's office. I sat up straight—I just corrected my posture as I write this—and waited for Mr. Turner to come into his office.

He walked in, sat down, and asked me in his southern accent, "Son, what do you know about my little company?" I was so thankful that I did the research. To this day, my mind is a blur as to what I actually said. I know I mentioned how his father started a billboard business, how Ted purchased a small UHF station—those of you who don't know what UHF is, Google it—how he created the superstation concept and believed that the right content would drive business and ad revenue.

After our conversation, Ted dismissed me, and I walked back to Carol's office. She told me that I would have an answer the following week.

I got the job! Ted hired me! Now came the decision, one of my major crossroads in life. Do I stick with the public sector or immerse myself in the private sector and work for one of the greatest visionaries in the media field? I chose the media. Since then, I have never looked back. Hence, I started one of the greatest jobs anyone could ever grow into, and on the personal side, this choice created a long career working side-by-side with my brother. What more could anyone ask?

And the adventure continues...

# 8: MOM'S DEATH

Death is that state in which one exists only in
the memory of others, which is why it is not
an end, no goodbyes, only good memories.
–Tasha Yar

Coming to terms with a loss is the most difficult task
we must face in our lives. Coming to terms with the
death of a parent is inexpressible. I will never forget
the day I received a call at work from our uncle, my
mother's brother.

"Andy, it's Mark." He said in his deep voice. Every
time he spoke, I was reminded, for some reason, of
Neil Diamond. He continued, "Your mom is getting
worse. The doctor's say pneumonia is in her lungs,
plus the complications from the MS are taking a toll
on her. They are not sure she will make it through
the night. I can't tell you what to do, but if I were
you, get down here quickly."

Our mom moved down to Florida with our
grandmother. Why? Because of the weather! Who
gets pneumonia in a state of the art nursing home in
Boca Raton, Florida!? To this day, I ask myself that
question.

I went and found my brother. Good thing we
worked on the same floor in the same tower at the
CNN center. He was on one end of the floor; I was on
the other. I walked into his office and closed the

door. It took all my strength not to start crying. Even as I write this, it is very hard not to. I explained the situation to him. I booked us on the first available flight to West Palm Beach early the following day. I called my uncle back and told him our arrival time, slightly past eleven the next morning. He said he would be at the airport to get us.

I didn't sleep that night; even if we jumped in a car and drove, it would take us ten hours to get there. The flight was going to be quicker. When we traveled together in those days, we always sat in the back of the plane. We sat together, but we did not talk. My brother got a drink and went to sleep. He, like me, did not sleep the night before.

Normally, we would talk about work and bro stuff, but not today. I knew my brother was trying to be strong, but he didn't like to show emotions outwardly. Neither did our father. I, on the other hand, had a hard time remaining stoic. I kept thinking, "Can't this plane go any faster? Why is the world not stopping? Our mom is sick; there should be no laughing, just get us to the airport and step-on-it!"

We land about an hour and a half later. We jumped up before the plane came to a complete stop, so we could gain some headway on disembarking the aircraft. As soon as we exited the plane and walked into the terminal, I heard my name over the intercom, "Andy Drooker, please pick up the red courtesy phone." I just look at my bro. We knew.

I picked up the phone; it was my uncle, "Andy, is Matthew with you?" he said.

"Yes. What is going on? Why aren't you here?" I asked with a tremble in my voice that alerted my brother; we knew before the words were spoken.

Our uncle continued, "We told your mom you were coming. She tried. She tried so hard to hold on till you both got here, but about thirty minutes ago, her lungs just stopped. She went—"

I hung up the phone. I could not hold it in any longer. I lost it at the airport. I dropped to my knees and just cried. I don't know how long I remained in that position. My brother hovered over me, like a shield, keeping people away from us. He walked in circles, saying, "It's not fair! It's not fair!"

Who am I to disagree with my bro? Our uncle found us, and honestly, I don't remember the trip to the nursing home. By the time we got there, her body was gone. Just the belongings in her room remained, her entire life in a room. Pictures of her family, my brother and I, during our years of growing up, hung on her walls and sat on her dresser. She kept all the stuffed animals we gave her. Her TV always played CNN, and she'd always say, "I never know if I might see either of you in the background. Ever since I saw you walk behind the anchors during the Gulf War and the OJ chase, I keep looking!" Matthew turned off the TV.

We both said, "Now what?"

Our uncle replied, "We need to pack-up her room. Not to sound morbid, but when someone passes-away no matter where people always come into the room and take belongings. Afterward, we will head to my place; you can stay there or at a hotel."

My brother and I borrowed our uncle's car, drove to Target, and purchased the largest piece of luggage we could find. We went back to our mom's room. Packing up a loved one's belongings is very, very hard. If anyone says otherwise, don't believe them.

For every little item each of us put in the luggage, we told a story about the when, where, and what. Who would have thought that every item in our mom's room had a story? But then again, everything and everyone has a story. We got everything into the luggage, turned to look at the room one more time, and left that nursing home for the last time, ever.

Matthew and I decided to stay in a hotel. We got one of those rooms that had a sitting room and a bedroom with two beds. We were told that the next day we had to go to the local funeral home and make the arrangements. Again another night with no sleep, thoughts flooded my mind. I kept thinking about stories of the recently deceased visiting their loved ones spiritually after death. Did I stay up secretly hoping I could see my mom again? Or was it grief that kept me awake?

Our uncle picked us up the next day and drove us to the funeral home. This was the first time I ever entered one as a client; it is very different going as a client rather than a guest. My brother and I were taken into a sterile room.

The representative of the funeral home explained that our mom would be sent to a home in Boston. She would be buried in the family lot next to her father, our grandfather. We discussed the cost of a casket, travel costs, permits, and other details. My brother put down his credit card and just said, "Whatever it takes, do it!"

I just looked at him, and he put his hand on my back and said, "Don't worry, Bro!"

After the paperwork was done, the representative asked us if we would like to say goodbye before she was sent to Boston. I just looked at my brother, tears in my eyes; he said, "Yes!"

We were led to a back room, and she was covered with a white sheet with her head exposed. My brother went over to her first. He kissed her forehead. He then turned to me and said, "She is so cold, are you sure you want to do this?"

I held back the tears and said, "Yes. This is the last time we will ever see her. I need to." I walked over. I bent down slowly. I put my lips to her head and started crying. I could not stop. "She's so cold, Bro!" said sobbing.

He pulled me away. My baby brother was my big brother. He took me out of there. The rest of the day, I was in twilight. I walked, people talked to me, but I was not in my body. I wanted to get out of that state so badly. I even thought about renting a car and just driving. The only solace I felt was knowing that when we left Florida the next day, our mom would be on the same plane with us. But she was on her way to Boston.

The next two days were a blur. I remember telling people I would not be at work. Everyone on my team and my boss, Larry, said they would go to Boston.

My brother and I arrived in Boston; it was the first time we had gone to Boston for something other than seeing our father. It was weird; fly-in, go to a funeral, fly-home. The day before the funeral, we met with the rabbi, who came out of retirement to preside over Mom's service. He was the same rabbi that presented at her bat mitzvah those many years ago—a bat mitzvah is an initiation ceremony for a Jewish girl of the age of twelve years and one day; it signifies she reached the age of religious maturity. When he heard about our mom, he contacted us and asked to lead the service. Telling a rabbi no does not occur that often. We welcomed it, and we're humbled and honored.

The day arrived. Matthew and I found the small cemetery. A tent was set up. Our mom's casket was off to the side. The rabbi asked us if we had anything we would like to put in the casket with her, as a reminder of her life with us and on God's earth. My brother put in a TV Guide and a letter. I put in a letter and a Snickers bar. Our mom loved reading the TV Guide and eating Snickers bars!

She always completed the TV Guide crossword puzzle. Little did she know, both her sons would go into media one day! At the graveside with us were friends, family, and our bosses from CNN. They flew in from New York and Atlanta to be with us. To this day, I cannot thank them enough for being part of our extended family. As I write this, I come to tears.

Never, never, I cannot express this enough, take anyone for granted. Life is a gift. Family is a gift. Friends are gifts. At any time, no one is immune to death. I implore you, if you get anything out of these words or this book, is treat each day as it could be your last. Tomorrow does not come with a guarantee.

People often ask the question, "If you could have anything in this world, what would you wish for?" People respond with cars, money, fame, fortune, women, men, and so on. Do not think of things; think of people. I would give anything, I mean anything, to hear and talk to my mother for five minutes. Treat yourself and your loved ones like life is not guaranteed because it is not!

When a person is young, everything is given to them. However, as that person ages, people, places, and things are taken away from them. Always remember those people. For if you do, they will always be with you in your heart and soul. I know that my loved ones accompany me on this journey. They are with me now, as I write this.

And the adventure continues...

# 9: BEV–INNER STRENGTH

When we meet real tragedy in life, we can react in two ways—either by losing hope and falling into self-destructive habits or by using the challenge to find our inner strength.
–Dalai Lama

Inner strength. We all have it. Maybe we just don't know it until we need it. Regardless, inner strength is not measured by the number of pull-ups you do, the number marathons you complete, or the number of hot dogs you eat in a fixed amount of time. Inner strength is something that is grown and nurtured; it tests you.

Inner strength sometimes has to be shown to you before you fully understand or comprehend how strong you have to be to overcome a roadblock. This roadblock is right in front of you on the road called life.

Many people have touched my heart in a way to awaken my sense of inner strength. But no one has done it as profoundly as Beverly "Bev" Beeson.

Bev was one of the strongest, bravest, and most courageous bosses I had the good fortune to meet on my journey. Her attitude and demeanor toward crisis, people, events, anything, never wavered. She was grace under pressure. Trust me, we had pressure at CNN. Just look at your history, starting with the

Gulf War. Every major world event, from shock and awe military campaigns to OJ Simpson's white Bronco, Bev and her team were responsible for ensuring that everything ran smoothly, from an operations perspective.

One cold and gray winter day, I was in Bev's office. Its position looked outside the CNN Center. From her office, you could see the U.S. Federal building, parking lots, and most of the buildings of the Georgia State University campus. Great view.

She called me into her office for an impromptu meeting and listed no subject on her invite. Attendance was mandatory. My mind started thinking, "Okay, what did I do?"

I admit it; I had a habit of doing things first, then asking for forgiveness afterward. Most of the time, this methodology worked well. I solved problems before they became a crisis. Although there were a few times where the word "Ooops!" would slip in the conversation. Trust me, "Ooops!" is not an excuse. It is a reason to question one's thinking—mainly mine.

So, this invitation got me thinking and thinking. I asked my team, "Hey, does anyone remember something I did recently that I, maybe, should have checked with Bev first?"

The response was an overwhelming, "No, not this week. Can't think of anything. Everything is running perfectly!"

"Thanks, everyone. Just wanted to check before my mandatory meeting with Bev." I replied.

Someone said, "I am sure it is nothing serious. Maybe it is just a check-in? You know Bev, if it were serious or urgent, she would have us and security find you!"

"You're right! She did that before. That was embarrassing for me when security came into the bathroom looking for me. Hey, no laughing. How would you like it if—never-mind." I said, walking away.

I made my way down to Bev's office. I had my notebook in tow, project status reports, and upcoming projects and trips to the international offices. I was as prepared as I could be. Boy, was I wrong!

I arrived at Bev's office doorway. She saw me in and then closed the door behind me. This is serious; Bev never closes her door. She always keeps one ear open as to what is going on. News events happen at any time, and her departments needed to be ready. She sat down in her executive chair directly across from me. A five-foot-tall world globe was to my left. Her wall of windows looking out over the city had the curtains drawn, the light was bright, but the mood was very serious. I sat up straight and listened.

"Andy, you know that you and your brother are the sons I never had. You both came here and were made part of this family, my family. You come up to my home anytime I have issues, we grab lunch, dinner and have spent many nights here during elections, news events, name it, we've seen it. We have seen the world change from our desks." I started to open my mouth; Bev put up her hand in a stopping position and continued, "I trust you and your brother implicitly. I want to share something with you. This is very hard for me, but the process of healing and acceptance must begin now. Also, you are now part of my support system. You always have been and will be there."

"Bev, are you okay? What's wrong? Is your family okay?" my voice cracked as the words escaped from my mouth.

Bev stood up, walked around her desk, and was now standing to my right. She raised her left arm, grabbed her hair, and with one quick jerk of her hand, pulled off her wig. I stood up. My eyes began to water—and do again as I write this. She hugged me. I don't know how long we stood together like that as tears rolled down my cheeks.

I had to regain my composure. This was Bev, one of the most powerful women in broadcasting at the time. She released me from our hug. I stepped back while wiping my eyes. Questions spiraled through my brain, but what is the etiquette for this? Bev just shared an incredibly personal and intimate aspect of her life. She had cancer. She chose to share this news with me, my brother, and a few other close colleagues. How does one react to this?

Bev returned to her seat behind her desk but left her wig off. The hair on her head was shaved like a marine. "Oh, you have no idea how good this feels. Those things are hot! They keep the heat in; my scalp can't breathe." She started laughing. I began to relax. She continued, "Being told one has cancer is not an easy pill to swallow. I went through so much emotional denial and anger. But I realized I don't have to do this alone. Yes, I have my family at home. But I have my family and support system here also. It was time to share, and it's okay. I, we, will make it through this. Having a disease does not make one unable to perform work. Sure, every other week, I have to do chemo on Fridays. That gives me the weekend to recoup from the therapy. You will see me at lunchtime walking around the atrium for exercise to keep my strength up. Or, you can do something so incredibly stupid, but genius, to get my blood pressure up. Come to think of it, that's a given, as sure as the sun sets and rises!" I laughed.

She continued, "Do not treat me like I am handicapped. Do not treat me any differently. Do not pity me. Do not feel sorry for me. This is the hand I have been dealt. I am in the game until the dealer says otherwise." She paused. "Now, tell me about this new system you want to deploy globally. It sounds like it could do away with—"

As I left her office, I did not feel sad. I felt honored, needed. I was just taught a life lesson. Bev illustrated courage, strength, and vulnerability all at once. What a role model for someone facing a continuous battle against their own body. Little did I know at the time, this event would help me have the same courage and fortitude for the journey ahead of me.

Bev fought the fight for twelve years. She kept coming to work; she kept things moving. Then one day after Christmas in 2008, the dealer called. Bev showed me that inner strength is a powerful weapon against anything. She was one of the strongest people I had the good fortune to meet and travel with on my journey. Bev, thank you for showing me a strength I did not know I had.

And the adventure continues...

# 10: LARRY G.–PERSEVERANCE

One of the advantages of being the captain, Doctor, is being able to ask for advice without necessarily having to take it.
–Captain James. T. Kirk

The task of the leader is to get his people from where they are to where they have not been.
–Henry Kissinger

During my life journey, I have been fortunate and honored to have met some extraordinary individuals. I've already introduced you to some of them. Larry, although he might not have known it at the time, had a profound effect on me and my ability to become an effective leader not just at Turner but throughout my career.

Larry and I started three weeks apart at Turner. In those days, the offices of Turner looked like an overstuffed closet that one pushed everything into, with the door barely able to close. The carpet had more duct tape holding it together then carpeting fibers. Those were the days of inspiration, drive, and determination to be the best.

Throughout our years at Turner, Larry became my boss, my mentor, and my friend. Over thirty years later, we can pick-up the phone and talk like no time has passed. He is now a grandfather, and I am a father. Time might have passed, but I will carry the lessons he instilled in me throughout my life. His words of wisdom on how to become an effective leader and innovator still ring true today. They are:

## NEVER STOP LEARNING
The more knowledge you have, the more creative you can be. The more you can do, the more solutions you have for problems.

## HAVE CO-WORKERS WITH DIFFERENT VIEWS
Weak leaders surround themselves with yes-men afraid to argue with them. That kind of leadership creates a team culture that stifles creativity and innovation. Worst of all, it keeps team members from speaking up due to fear of retaliation.

## ALWAYS BE PART OF YOUR TEAM
When you are in a leadership role, it is easy to let yourself get away from leading. Sure, with leadership comes perks. Nice office. An assistant to help with day-to-day activities, etc. Every day is filled with meetings and decisions to be made. It is easy to trap yourself in the office and forget what is happening on the front-lines. When a leader loses that perspective, it is harder to understand what the team is doing and the best ways to solve problems. The bottom line, when you are not involved with your team, it is easy to lose their trust and have them complain about how you, as their leader, do not understand their job.

## PLAY POKER, NOT CHESS

Who doesn't like chess? However, chess is often taken too seriously as a metaphor for leadership strategy. For all its intricacies, chess is a game defined by rules that can be predicted. It is a game of boxes and limitations. Poker is a better analogy for strategy. Life is a game of probabilities, not defined by rules. Often understanding the landscape of competitors is a much greater advantage than the cards you have in your hand. Bluffs, tells, and bets are all a big part of a real-life strategy. Playing that strategy, with an eye always on the competition, often leads to better outcomes than following the rigid rules of chess. That is the key, don't follow the rigid rules, because you will find yourself in a limited box.

An example of the above mentoring advice came into play when the corporate IT department insisted the whole company be on one unified email system. I vocally disagreed. I made the argument to Larry that the proposed system would not enable ad sales to communicate in different languages, which utilized double-byte characters—languages like Japanese and Chinese, for example. From a business strategy, this would greatly limit the ad sales teams in certain parts of the world from communicating with the necessary business etiquette.

For example, if Turner Broadcasting acts as a gaijin, outsider company, in Japanese business, we will be treated as such. However, if we take the time to communicate in the native language, our entrance into that international market would be more widely accepted. It would help our employees working in the

Tokyo office remain effective when communicating with local ad agencies.

Larry requested a proposal for this global endeavor. I presented it in person. His response, behind closed doors, was, "This is your area of expertise. I have never questioned your wisdom or recommendations. I am going to approve this for all the ad sales offices around the world. However—" I stopped him there.

"Larry, if this is the wrong direction for ad sales, I will resign. No excuses! I believe this is the correct path strategically, and it is the future direction for the company." I left his office and started the deployment of this new mail system around the world for ad sales.

That system, in beta at the time, was Microsoft Exchange, which is now the global leader in email systems.

Think outside the boxes and limitations, and a whole world is open to possibilities. Thank you, Larry, for opening my eyes.

And the adventure continues...

# 11: HOW DID I GET HERE? THE FIRST DATE

When you are courting a nice girl, an hour seems like a second. When you sit on a red-hot cinder, a second seems like an hour. That's relativity.
–Albert Einstein

It was the year 2011. I happily worked at The Weather Channel. Every aspect of my life seemed to be going well, except I had no one to share it with me. Surprisingly, my health was doing well; my asthma was under my control, and I practiced yoga to reduce residual pain from the spinal fusion I had in 2009.

While speaking with a friend, she suggested I try a matchmaking service. At first, I thought, "Am I that undesirable that I cannot find a life-mate on my own?" No, that was not it. It was not me; it was, in my opinion, society.

As technology developed, our society changed. The rules of dating also changed. Sure, I could go on one of the many dating websites, write a profile, and put myself out there. Well, I am not ashamed to admit it, but I tried that. And you know what I found? The same people were on all the various dating websites. Also, I unfortunately discovered, everyone lies! This truly discouraged me. So, I figured what do I have to lose except money and time. It is not like I am in a race. I just wanted what everyone wants, happiness and a family.

Ultimately I was introduced to a wonderful dating coach and adviser. She took my case and made it her personal responsibility to find me a woman, and not just a woman, "The Right Woman."

The process continued for months, yes, you read that right, months. I met some interesting and wonderful women, and with some of them, I felt I had a connection. I dated one particular woman for a few months; we talked regularly and spent our free time together. Sometimes I sent her flowers, just because.

Then, suddenly, she went dark. No explanation, nothing. She contacted the matchmaker and canceled her membership. Unfortunately, this took me back to square one. Not only did I spend months dating this woman, my "happily ever after" woman could have gotten away while I was otherwise occupied.

I did not waste time wondering what I did wrong, if anything, nor let it affect my self-esteem. I jumped right back into the ocean. Then the matchmaker presented me with two wonderful Jewish women—one worked in media at CNN, and one worked at Coke. My parents always wanted me to meet a nice Jewish girl. In the end, though, they just wanted me to be happy. So, the matchmaker set up dinner dates with each of them.

Date night came to meet the woman from Coke. She was a goddess, or what I thought a goddess should look like. Firm, curves packed into a tight body. Her hair was a cascade of lustrous brown curls bouncing gently off her shoulders down her back. Her eyes were shimmering blue pools that you ached to dive into. From her moist, shiny lips came a gentle voice, flavored with a slight accent, both exotic and musical. "Andy?"

I felt like I was hearing my name for the first time. "Andy," I thought to myself, "you are having the best dream of your life." Unfortunately, that dream ended, but not by my choice. Her name was Lorelei, otherwise known as the siren.

In my eyes, the evening was wonderful. The conversation was excellent and flowed easily; we had many things in common, including life-dreams and aspirations. We both wanted a family.

The next day the matchmaker informed me that she had a good time and wanted to go out again. I was sold on this woman. But, the matchmaker told me that I still had another date at the end of the week. It was a l-o-n-g week. I kept thinking about Lorelei. I thought, "How can I go out on a date with someone else when I wanted to focus my energies on just one woman?" I committed to meet woman number two. Besides, one never knows what might happen. Or not.

Woman number two was already seated when I arrived at the restaurant. She was beautiful. Her eyes were like windows to her soul; her blond curly hair appeared to float on her shoulders. Her attitude and demeanor were so inviting that all my worries seem to melt away. Our time at the restaurant seemed to fly by. It was closing time, and we still talked. We had similar goals, likes, and hobbies. She enjoyed photography, worked in media, and was so very likable and attractive. Before the evening was over, we set our next date for the following weekend. Her name was Nadia.

Meanwhile, Lorelei was on an international trip with her brother. However, during the trip, she and I exchanged emails. She told me that there were more women than men on the trip, and her brother was the object of attraction by many possible suitors. Over email, we planned our second date upon her return.

During the week, I spoke to Nadia on the phone, and we began to develop a connection. She was so easy to talk with. She shared some of her photography with me, and I was impressed. I offered to set up a website for her and advised her to purchase her own domain name. When she did this, I knew she trusted my advice and listened to what I had to say. I looked forward to our second date with anxious anticipation.

The second date night with Nadia arrived. I picked her up at her home, and we headed to the restaurant. We had a wonderful evening; as we finished our dinner, it was getting late, and she suggested we leave the establishment before they kicked us out like on our first date. I took her home, and she invited me in to see her condo. Who was I to say no! Our conversation continued where it left at the restaurant.

Now, this is where I realized the saying, "It's a small world," is so true. As Nadia talked, I noticed some books on her kitchen counter; they were books on dating. I asked why she needs dating advice books, and she told me they were from her ex-boyfriend's sister.

The sister had them, but now that her brother had broken up with Nadia, she thought Nadia might find them useful. She dropped them off just before leaving on an international trip with her brother. One can imagine what is starting to go through my mind. No way! There is no way that Lorelei and Nadia know each other on that close of a personal level. Never mind, was I a rebound date for Nadia?

As the evening continued, I kept this revelation to myself. However, Nadia was getting physically closer and closer to me. I mentioned that it was getting late, and I should be heading home.

To my surprise, but a tremendous boost to my self-esteem, before I touched the doorknob, Nadia pinned me against the wall and kissed me passionately. She did not let up. It seemed like the kiss went on for an eternity. She released me with the promise to fully continue where we left off on our next date, which she wanted to be the next day.

I immediately called the matchmaker. The thoughts going through my mind were mixed. I was angry, embarrassed, and turned on all at the same time. But yet, I felt dirty. Why, you might ask? Because, during this date with Nadia, I was thinking about Lorelei. Wrong I know, but my heart was somewhere else.

I did not have any more contact with Nadia after that evening. The matchmaker played the bad-guy, and I then focused all my energies on Lorelei.

At the time, I thought I made the right decision. Did Lorelei feel the same emotions about me as I did her? Or, did I just meet the criteria on a checklist? Only time would tell.

And the adventure continues...

# 12: THE COURTSHIP–THE NEXT SIX MONTHS

After a time, you may find that having is not so pleasing a thing, after all, as wanting. It is not logical, but it is often true.
–Commander Spock

In self–reflection regarding the courtship, I realized something that many of my friends and family had tried telling me, "You are a checklist." I came along at the right time when Lorelei wanted to get engaged, married, then have children.

On November 22, 2011, I asked Lorelei's father for permission to marry his daughter, and we became engaged almost a month later on December 23, 2011. We married on May 6, 2012. Our miracle daughter was born in December 2012. Approximately three years later, we were divorced.

Neither the CF nor being a caregiver was on Lorelei's checklist. To this day, when I review those three years, Sydney is the only positive thing I look back on with pride. The only exception is the personal growth I embraced during my medical journey, a journey supported by many others and not my then–wife.

Upon further review of my journals, not once, during my entire medical journey, did Lorelei say, "I love you. I am here for you."

It should also be noted that even now, as I write this, Lorelei forbids me to speak to or communicate with Sydney's only living grandparents. That fact in itself says a lot regarding the control and manipulation I lived with during my marriage. I was convenient, nothing more, nothing less. How very sad. It explains much of the darkness I was in. But does not excuse it.

I always wanted a family, children. This is the dream of millions of single people. But, as I learned the hard way, the quote opening this chapter is so very true, at least for me. The adage, "If it sounds too good to be true, it probably is," is not always correct. However, in this instance, it was. I saw what I wanted to see, not what was there. The first signpost was when she asked for a three-carat diamond ring, a few months into dating.

And the adventure continues...

# 13: THE MEDICAL ROAD MAP– JOURNEY TAKEN

Prescription: A physician's guess at what will best prolong the situation with least harm to the patient.
–Ambrose Bierce

They certainly give very strange names to diseases.
–Plato

## AUGUST 2013

There I was, leaving the doctor's office with the words, "six months to live" and "lung transplant" replaying over and over in my head.

I headed home to tell Lorelei. She was concerned, however, not so much about my health, but more about our insurance coverage. Rightly so. She was six months pregnant with our miracle child. My only course of action was to go into work the next day, contact HR/benefits, and start the process to be issued the short term disability (STD) forms needed for my doctor to complete.

While speaking to the representative regarding my illness and the process of STD, the HR rep's demeanor and attitude were unsympathetic and cold. It felt like I was being reprimanded and interrogated for even requesting this benefit. This was the first, but certainly not the last doubting attitude I encountered on my medical journey. By the end of the day, I was on thirty-day STD, dependent upon the benefits center receiving all the documentation from my physician.

## SEPTEMBER 2013

I had been on oxygen for a month.

Oddly, my first destination on this journey was with a nutritionist. Normally, people go to nutritionists if they have diabetes, heart disease, are overweight, or have some sort of problem relating to eating or digestion. The nutritionist I saw told me that I was the first patient she'd instructed to eat anything, and as much of it, as possible. My goal? Gain weight, period. I told her that's what I'd done my entire life, and I asked her what I should change.

"Go to Waffle House, daily," was her response. A scientific and nutritious answer. At that moment, I knew I had a long road ahead! The problem was, my brain and heart were still in the go-gear, and I began to feel like all this medical advice was bullshit.

The next stop was Emory Healthcare for lung transplant evaluation. I was assigned to Dr. Staton, who is now retired. I found him to be stand-offish; I knew from his attitude and demeanor he was skeptical regarding my need for a lung transplant. In fact, he questioned if I was even ill.

He decided to ignore all previous testing and subjected me to various expensive and painful tests. Much to his surprise, my Pulmonary Function Test (PFT) confirmed a decrease in my lung function for someone of my age and relatively good health. He then did what every previous doctor did—put me on steroids. One of the painful and expensive tests mentioned above was a bronchoscopy—it's like a colonoscopy for your lungs. All I could do is wait for the results.

A week later, the results came back. A sample of mucus taken from deep inside my lungs was growing—It's Alive! However, it was too early to determine what it was growing into. This further corroborated the original doctor's diagnosis; something was causing my lungs to lose capacity. At the same time, my white blood cell count went up, which signified I now fought battles on two fronts, the physical and psychological.

The initial thirty days for my STD passed. My primary doctor filled out forms monthly to help me get coverage for up to one-hundred-twenty days. That was the maximum for STD. Would it be enough? I did not consult the Magic-8-Ball on this question. At this rate, I already knew the answer.

## OCTOBER 2013

I now approached sixty days of STD. Dr. Staton called me and said, "You have an infection in your lungs; it could be tuberculosis (TB). We need a CAT scan. In the meantime, I am going to prescribe three drugs for you to take. However, they all have serious side-effects."

"How serious?" I asked, with a slight tremble in my voice.

"Loss of hearing, loss of eye-sight, and permanent liver damage." He responded in an uninflected voice.

What could I do? He wasn't even sure I had TB. However, if I did, and I didn't take the drugs, my journey might end before my daughter was born. At that point, I felt like I was falling deeper into a black hole. How deep? No light escapes a black hole, that deep!

Lorelei, pregnant with our daughter, had yet to accompany me on a doctor visit, nor had she spoken to me about how I was feeling or doing. Her focus, as it should be, was with our unborn daughter. She was completely uninterested in my emotional state. Thoughts of not being present at my daughter's first birthday flooded my mind. I felt alone in my own home. I turned to my mentor and second father, John.

## OCTOBER–DECEMBER 2013

I was treated for TB. My primary doctor disagreed with the diagnosis and referred me to an infectious disease specialist, Dr. Robin Dretler. John took me to my first appointment.

At this point, TB drugs were starting to harm me. I was getting weaker. After the initial exam and review of all the charts and records, Dr. Dretler referred me to National Jewish Health in Denver, Colorado.

A week later, my greatest accomplishment was born. I became a dad! The year ended on a high note!

## JANUARY 2014

In the first week of January, John and I went back to Dr. Dretler. He changed my overall diagnosis from TB to bronchiectasis, thus instigating a change to all my meds.

The second week of January was even more exciting. John and I headed to Denver for a full week of tests at National Jewish; subsequently, my diagnosis was changed to bronchiectasis and mycobacterium avium complex (MAC).

Now, with this different diagnosis, verified by several doctors at National Jewish, I was instructed to choose which hospital, in the southeast, I wanted to re-evaluate me for candidacy for a lung-transplant. I chose Duke Health.

Shortly after our return to Atlanta from Colorado, John and I headed to Duke Pulmonary for a day of evaluation and treatment. I was now officially a candidate—on the list—for a lung transplant.


## FEBRUARY 2014

Back in Atlanta, Sydney was two months old. The short term disability was officially over, which instigated the following: I must officially switch to long-term disability, I had to apply for social security, and I had to get a Medicare health plan. All sounds simple enough, right? Not even close.

This process taught me a life lesson regarding labels. During this entire process, no one mentioned that once you are labeled disabled and receive social security and Medicare benefits, if you decide, with your doctor, to go back into the workforce and decline social security and Medicare benefits, that you can't get back onto these benefits until retirement age.

In 2019 the requirements evolved. However, these requirements do not give recipients incentives to go back into the workforce. From a solely economic perspective related to health care, it implied that it is economically advantageous to keep your disabled status/label.

This fact alone would not motivate anyone to try to go back into the workforce. It meant to me that society gave up on me. I felt labeled a burden to society and my family. Why should I try to get well if I couldn't live something close to the life I had? How could I provide a future for my daughter if I was stuck in the disabled category, with no hope of crawling out of an ever-deepening hole?

Unknown to me, Lorelei was already discussing, with friends and family, about leaving me. I began to think of her as a siren, luring me in with her beauty and graciousness, eventually casting me off after I no longer served her needs. How could I have known when we got married, two years prior, that I would be on this journey? How could I face this alone without support from my spouse? This revelation would make anyone fall deeper into unbearable despair.

## MAY 2014

May brought a major milestone, our second wedding anniversary. The siren did not want to celebrate. From what I could see, she didn't take a single photo of us. However, I did find all the cards and letters I'd ever sent her in a box in the garage, marked trash. This was another signpost on the road; it further frayed my already fragile mental state.

I realized that I not only fought for my life, but I also fought to be with my daughter. She needed to know her dad. Never, at any time, did I think about giving her up. Even at the tender age of six months, she was a greater inspiration than the relationship that produced her. It didn't matter what drugs were prescribed; she inspired me to rethink my treatment.

I decided to practice yoga to help with my breathing and chronic back pain. I switched to eating all organic foods. Meanwhile, my lung function scores fell. At that point, only one doctor suggested that my back pain medication, fentanyl, might be causing or masking some of my symptoms.

John took me to the pain clinic I worked with since my spinal fusion in 2009. I requested to have my dosage reduced.

Their response was, "You want to decrease your pain meds. Why?"

After a lengthy discussion of my current medical state, they agreed to decrease my dosage, but in six-month increments. At that rate, I would be off the pain medication in two years. The timeline was not satisfactory. But, if I didn't decrease the dosage correctly, my body would not create its natural pain-fighting chemicals.

Here's an important safety tip to anyone out there who wants to get off pain meds; under no circumstances stop cold turkey. Work with your doctor; some methodologies work. It might take time, but in the end, you will be better for it. 'Nuff said!

## JULY 2014

I was back at Emory Healthcare, with Dr. Staton. My PFT was stable. This was an improvement; it was no longer falling. A small victory, but at this point, any win was cause for celebration. I knew that practicing yoga helped me control my breathing. I truly believe an exercise called "The Breath of Fire" helped me slowly get off oxygen in a tank to room air. My yoga instructor suggested acupuncture. Sure, why not, she hadn't been wrong yet.

## AUGUST 2014

Dr. Dretler now hypothesized I had an immune deficiency. My frustration moved from simmer to boil. "What the fuck?" I vented to John. We were now at the two-year mark on the journey, and still, no conventional medical treatment is working. I was barely stable on my PFT's. I was getting angry. The doctors followed a roadmap. Every road taken had a dead-end.

John and I went back to Dr. Degryse, the original doctor who started me down this path. She knows I am frustrated, sad, depressed, and have a non-supportive siren at home with an eight-month-old daughter, who was now in daycare. I was alone at home during the days. I received daily calls from John and his family and my brother. We decided to head back to Duke.

## SEPTEMBER 2014

John and I returned to Duke Health, and I received a whole new medical team. I was still on the transplant candidate list. I should be happy; a new set of lungs may mean a possible fresh breath at life.

I had a deep discussion with John; I was on the verge of giving up. The siren shared my home but remained stand-offish.

John took me back to Dr. Degryse. I wanted to take myself off the transplant list. Just give up. Why not? Why am I fighting when the siren does not even care if our daughter knows her father.

John and Dr. Degryse both said, "We are not giving up on you."

I broke down, "It is so hard. I feel like I am on this road by myself, and I keep hitting dead-ends. Do you know how that feels? One disappointment after another? What the hell is wrong with me? What the fuck is going on with my body? My daughter needs her father. She needs my yin to the siren's yang. She needs to know me, not just stories of me."

I don't know how long my emotional outburst lasted; I just remember looking up at John, wiping my face, and saying, "Sorry."

Dr. Degryse states, "We are all missing something."

I think to myself, "No, shit!"

She said she would contact Duke and get me back in there.

## NOVEMBER 2014
Sydney's first Thanksgiving.

## DECEMBER 2014
I caught the flu and landed in the hospital for a few days. Not what I needed.

## MARCH 2015
I was back at Duke Health, having my first meeting with the lung transplant team. I endured more painful and expensive tests.

I just have to state, for the record, the most painful test I'd had, up to this point, was the arterial blood gases test. You have been warned. It doesn't help that I hate needles, but, OMG, I would rather watch whole seasons of bad 80s TV shows than get that test again!

Guess what! My diagnosis changed again! Yep, now they said I had chronic obstructive pulmonary disease (COPD). New meds. All the old meds, thrown out. I asked the unanswerable question, "What damage did those meds do to me if I did not have the illness they were prescribed to treat?"

"That is a great question. Keep us informed as to any loss of vision or hearing, or if your eyes start turning yellow, which is a sign of liver damage." The lead doctor calmly stated.

I completed all the forms for getting moved from the lung transplant candidate list to the recipient list. This meant I would get a new set of lungs. As I write this, it is hard to fathom. Someone dies, I am on a list for their lungs.

The next appointment at Duke was set for late August or early September 2015. That appointment was the final week-long evaluation for transplant before receiving new lungs. I talked to doctors who evaluated my mental and physical state. I completed forms and more forms—just an FYI, there are more forms and processes getting lungs then I care to go into. I hope that those of you reading this never have to experience this process. What I will say is that the forms were depressing to read. The statistics they provided to help individuals make informed decisions were not promising—I am a data scientist—and I found them to be emotionally disconcerting.

## JULY–AUGUST 2015

The absentee siren took Sydney to see her grandparents. I was left at home, not invited. "I can't take care of you and Sydney while traveling."

The signposts were getting more frequent. Too bad. It turned out while I looked at a GPS, I missed reading the signs.

## AUGUST–SEPTEMBER 2015

Well, today was a big day. I drove to Duke by myself. No caregiver. John was ill. The siren didn't want to make the trip with me, her excuse long forgotten. However, it clearly illustrated, she did not want the title of caregiver.

So, I headed out alone to discover my fate—new lungs or something else. At that point, it was in God's hands. Or to be more precise, doctor's who thought they were gods.

I arrived at seven-thirty in the morning and was directed to the new-transplant-patient-orientation. At first, I was denied access because I didn't have a caregiver with me. After explaining that my caregiver could not attend, the staff contacted John by phone to verify that he was, indeed, my caregiver, and I was allowed to participate.

The post-op process was outlined clearly. All transplant recipients must stay within five miles of the hospital and treatment facilities for three months post-transplant. When you think about it, you'll realize a recipient of new lungs must learn how to breathe, walk, run, and exercise again, as well as take a regiment of daily medication to prevent infection and organ rejection. The medication alone per month could cost more than $3500.

If a recipient caught a common cold, it could mean a lengthy hospital stay or an infection leading to death. I asked myself, is this how I want my daughter to grow up? Having her father never to be able to go to her school or take her to Disneyland?

Up to this point, due to the siren, I was a father who was deliberately and systematically omitted from any external activities with his daughter. What would happen to my ability to independently participate in her life if I received a transplant?

I realized the siren had already given up on me when she asked, "Are all your affairs in order? Is your life insurance current?" Not very encouraging words.

As the evaluation week continued, I had a psychological evaluation, insurance verification, family finance verification, tests to determine tissue type, blood type, and many documents to sign. I felt like I was closing on a new house!

The day came when I met the surgical team that would perform the actual transplant. I met three surgeons.

The first surgeon came in, very staunch and serious. He introduced himself as the primary surgeon. His opening statement was, "First, I will cut you open, then I'll gut your chest cavity like a fish!" Honestly, I lost him at "cut you open!" I kept on thinking about all the times our father took us fishing on the thirteenth hole at Pinebrook. After he left, I felt more ill from our conversation than I felt from my condition.

The second surgeon came in. He, too, was serious but not so buttoned up. He wore blue scrubs and sneakers. His conversation revolved around the post-operative procedures and processes. He saw I was getting a little green in the face. His comment was, "If you cannot handle hearing about it, you most certainly cannot handle going through it." I tended to agree with his assessment. The pain and learning to breathe again at times would be frustrating but would pass with a lot of work and physical therapy. I was not afraid of the work, just the quality of life and the image my daughter would have of her father.

The third surgeon, the chief of staff, came in. He, too, wore blue scrubs and sneakers, but his demeanor seemed like that of Hawkeye Pierce from MASH. He proceeded to sit down at the small desk in the room, put his feet on the table, and said, "Son, something about your case does not add up. You are almost fifty, have gone through your entire life with asthma, and then unexpectedly, your oxygen saturation levels suddenly drop to the eightieth percentile. Each doctor you have seen has given you a different explanation, but no one has looked at the possible underlying causes. What caused the MAC? What is now causing you, a man in his forties, to be diagnosed with COPD? We are all missing the cause.

Then the single question came; the question that changed the course of this journey, "Have you ever been tested for CF?"

"What's CF?" I replied as I raised my shoulders up and down.

"Cystic fibrosis," he quickly responded. "Have you ever been tested?"

"Honestly, I don't know. Both my parents have passed. I know in recent days, CF was never mentioned. What's the test?"

"Normally, the test, which has been around since the 1950s, is given to children when they are about three years old. Basically, we make the patient sweat, collect the sweat, and then check it for a certain amount of chloride in the collected sweat. If you have greater then a certain amount of chloride, you have CF. Does this sound familiar?"

"Nope, never been tested."

"Okay, this is what I want to do. Just to cover all our bases, I would like to schedule you for a CF test tomorrow at the children's hospital. Wait here; I am going to get the scheduling group to do this right now."

Doctor three quickly left the room, came back within five minutes, and continued, "Be at the children's hospital across the street at nine tomorrow morning. They will run four tests on you. Then come back here the following day for the results. Scheduling will send you an email through the patient portal as to what time I can meet you," he finished.

"Thank you, doctor; I will see you in two days." I shook his hand; he opened the exam room door and escorted me to check-out.

I called the siren that night, thinking that she would want to hear the latest progress, or perhaps might want to know how the day went. She put Sydney on video so I could see her. My daughter was happier to see her daddy than the siren was to hear from her husband. After I said good night to my daughter, the siren seemed uninterested in this possible new and treatable diagnosis.

I said goodnight, and I tried calling my bro, but he was busy with work. I called John and his wife, Carol. John apologized for not being with me, but I told him to focus on getting better and that I would let them know the results of the test.

I was up early the next day, eager to get to the children's hospital. I ate well in the morning, still trying to gain weight. The drive to the hospital took less than five minutes; I parked the car and walked to the designated floor. After arrival and registration, I waited for my name to be called. Like most people, I brought reading material, just in case I had to wait. A little more than an hour passed.

I calmly walked up to the registration desk and asked if I was in the correct department. A nurse who stood behind the receptionist heard my name. The nurse stepped forward and spoke, "We are so sorry you had to wait this long. Honestly, we were looking for a four-year-old male, not a forty-nine-year-old male. We thought the chart had a mistake. To be honest, we have never tested anyone as old as you before."

"I will take that as a compliment," I replied with a smile and little laugh.

She proceeded to walk me down a long hallway with pictures of Muppets, Captain America, Iron Man, Superman, and Wonder Woman. Well, at least I was in good company. I did not tell them I had a Wonder Woman Graphic Novel in my backpack. I knew I was in the right place!

"If you can just wait here, we need to put two beds together since you are much taller than our normal patient." She said with a wonderfully large grin on her face.

"No problem," I replied.

As she put the beds together, I glanced around the wing of the hospital; it consisted entirely of children who had CF. All these children were between the ages of three and nine, and they were all isolated in their rooms, watching TV, playing video games, or reading.

I noticed the lack of a community room, and signs everywhere stated that all patients needed to stay at least five feet apart from each other. I asked why. The nurse told me that CF patients could get each other sick just by breathing on each other.

I was slowly getting an education on a disease that had been around for decades, yet I was being tested for it, forty-six years after I should have been.

After she finished setting up the beds, the nurse told me to get comfortable because I was going to be in the same position for a few hours. Once I was situated, she and another nurse piled blankets on me and turned on heat lamps, all in the name of instigating sweating. After my temperature started to rise, she told me to roll-up both shirt sleeves to expose my forearms.

After telling me it wouldn't hurt, she started the initial sweat collection processes on my right arm. The first step was to put a chemical, pilocarpine, on my skin. Then she wrapped an electrode around my arm, covering the area where the chemical was applied. Next, after she could see sweat, she removed the electrode and collected the sweat on filter paper gauze. She needed to collect a minimal amount for the test to be accurate.

She completed the test twice on each arm. After a few hours, I was free to go back to the hotel to rest. I thanked them for accommodating an older patient, such as myself. They laughed and wished me the best.

Needless to say, I was in a fog for the rest of the day. Before I went back to the hotel, I stopped off at Whole Foods to pick up dinner. I brought it back to my room, finished it, and got ready for bed. I called the siren and received the same treatment as the night before. I felt almost like I was inconveniencing her by calling to tell her about my day and requesting to see my baby girl.

All these signposts and I was still blind. I talked to my brother. He said, "No way. Mom would have had you tested." I agreed with him. He closed the call out, letting me know he will be there for me. "Don't worry, Bro," he said in his deep monotone voice. My baby brother never worries about anything. He rolls with it. I am blessed to have him as a brother. I could not reach John.

It was my last day at Duke. Either I have CF, or the original diagnosis was correct, and I need a lung transplant to live. Hawkeye walked into the patient room. Assumed his previous position with his feet on the desk and then bluntly stated, "Son, you have CF. Your chloride test result was 62– 65.9. Anything over 60 is a positive marker for CF. We tested you four times. I've never met any of your other doctors, but all the signs were there.

I cannot begin to imagine the roller coaster you have been on for the past two years. But, at least now, we can treat you for the correct disease. However, although this might be good news, there is always bad news. The bad news here is the disease, like the house, always wins. But, with proper treatment, you can lead a normal but maybe, limited life. Listen to me when I say this; you have beaten the odds. You have lived all forty-nine years with a disease that normally—" he trailed off, and then continued, "and did you know the majority of CF males cannot conceive children? I understand you are a new father. If your daughter has your will power and the strength you have shown, she is one lucky girl." His words echoed in my mind even after he stopped.

"Okay, so what I heard was I don't have MAC, asthma, or TB?" I asked with a slight tremble in my voice.

"Son, I don't think you ever had asthma or any of those other diseases your other doctors diagnosed you with. I believe that one or a combination of the medications you were on since you were three kept you alive all these years. You have accomplished a lot for someone who should have died in their teens. You are, at least for me, the oldest living patient with CF that I have had the good fortune of treating without having to cut into.

At some point, will you need new lungs, maybe? Do you need them now? No. Let's get you connected to a CF doctor and properly treat you. After forty-nine years, you are due for the correct medication."

I walked out of my final day at Duke with a revitalized sense of self, a new sense of life. Maybe I would see my daughter graduate high school, give her away at her wedding, be a grandfather.

John was beyond happy, although, sometimes with him, it is hard to tell.

My bro enthusiastically said, "I knew you never had all that other shit. Maybe doctors should read WebMD more. The facts just did not fit the situation."

The siren's response, "That is great news, does this mean I don't have to take care of you anymore? Did the doctor mention when can you go back to work?"

A week after this major great news, the siren left for Toronto on a trip with her parents and brother with Sydney in tow. She felt it would have been too much of an inconvenience to travel with me and the possible oxygen tanks I might need.

I saw a signpost ahead, but couldn't quite read it. What does it say?

## MARCH 2016

I went back to Duke Health three times after the momentous diagnosis.

The first was in March 2016. Duke referred me to the Emory CF Clinic. I now had a local CF doctor that prescribed medication—Pulmozyme and saline solution—to treat the CF. These two medications work together to clear the breathing airways. However, the doctors at Duke didn't believe that these improved my breathing as well as they should.

However, on the side of good news, my gastro-enterologist figured out, before the CF diagnosis, that a pancreatic enzyme deficiency caused my weight loss. He put me on the drug Creon. This drug helped my pancreas break-down nutrients in food more effectively and enabled me to gain weight. It should be noted that the majority of CF patients are on Creon. Another signpost missed.

It was at this point in my journey that the use of fentanyl was discussed at length between my doctors and me. As I mentioned previously, I had been on the drug since 2009. Eventually, I realized that fentanyl, besides killing the physical pain I experienced from the spinal fusion, also killed the pain of everything else—a failing marriage, a change in lifestyle, living with the label of being disabled, not being able to provide for the siren or our daughter.

Keep in mind, I loved my family, but in my thoughts, I was a poor husband and a poor father. I was deeply depressed. I received absolutely no encouragement from the siren, who was supposed to be my rock, not hurl them at me.

The doctor firmly instructed that I must get off fentanyl if I wanted any hope of recovery, as it could be masking other symptoms. Also, if I decided that I wanted a lung transplant, I had to be opioid-free.

In the current world of pain management for post-operative pain, only in extreme cases are opioids utilized.

This might seem like an easy hurdle to overcome; just stop wearing the medicated patch. Right? No. Weaning myself off fentanyl was the hardest action I had to take to get to the tomorrows I wanted.

Was I addicted to the absence of emotional and physical pain? Yes, yes, I was. Why experience pain? Because pain defines you. It makes you realize what you are fighting for. Fighting gives you motivation and gives you hope. Fighting makes you realize or rediscover your purpose. Most of all, in my case, I wasn't just fighting for myself; I was fighting for loved ones.

Let me be perfectly clear, removing any gray area; I would sacrifice anything for my loved ones—including the siren, but as mentioned previously, she was already talking to friends and family about leaving me, but never to me. No matter what I did, I had to face the hard truth that she would no longer be in my life. No matter how much I fought, she already left my corner.

# AUGUST 2016

It was time for my second return visit to Duke since my CF diagnosis. This was the last time the siren accompanied me. She brought Sydney, who was now two, along with her. To this day, I have no idea why they came with me to that appointment. She was inattentive while the doctor reviewed my latest test results.

I gave my doctor the latest update. I used oxygen only when needed, mostly at night. My PFT numbers improved. I started decreasing the use of fentanyl. As alternatives to opioids, I utilized Biofeedback, new relaxing exercises to control my breathing, as well as therapeutic massage therapy. But the greatest accomplishment, which garnered the most significant results, was attending physical therapy instead of pulmonary rehab. This decision was a true game-changer for my health.

First and foremost, my physical therapist, Steve, took it upon himself to work holistically with me. Not just on exercise, but nutrition, cardio, and physical therapy for my back pain. All of these factors were far more effective physically than any of the drugs I had taken. Treat and feed your body correctly, and it will start following the correct path. The key was being dedicated to and maintaining the regimen Steve outlined for me while finding and sustaining balance. The adage, "No pain, no gain," is fiction.

He taught me that if I felt pain, two things were happening. First, my body was acclimating to the decreased levels of fentanyl, and second, my body was beginning to communicate correctly to my brain that something was right or wrong. In this instance, the pain was an identifier of getting well, not getting sicker.

The best news was the oxygen saturation levels in my blood were now greater than ninety-five percent on room air with no supplemental oxygen!

My doctor at Duke felt that with this level of breathing improvement, positive test results, and the new regimen of physical therapy, I was still a satisfactory candidate for a lung transplant. However, it was too early to consider it!

My actions, taking control, and owning my wellness plan, contradictory to the norm, had a vastly positive effect on my mind, body, and spirit. Everyone in my corner, barring the one person who took a vow to always be there, was ecstatic for my accomplishment. Yet amid these successes, the end of my marriage was closer then I realized.

## LATE 2016–NOW

The next visit to Duke was scheduled for February 2017. Before that date, the siren filed for divorce. Sydney was just over three years old. She will never remember when Mommy and Daddy lived together as a family. The siren had already moved on.

Depression crept back. The darkness returned with a vengeance. I fought and fought to get well for myself, my daughter, and what I perceived as a family. But it was a facade put up over three years.

Again I wondered what I was fighting for. Then I realized my tomorrows, whether they number one, ten, one hundred or one thousand—anything greater than zero—was a gift. A gift like that should be cherished and fought for. And, I do treasure them every minute of every day.

It was, is, and always shall be about Sydney. She is my legacy to the world. She is aware that a father's love knows no bounds. I can only hope she sees that her unconditional love, admiration for, and belief in her daddy (DaDa) motivated him and pushed him to "fly like a butterfly and sting like a bee." Sydney helped me win round after round against an illness with horrible odds. She helped me stay strong when my cornerman left my corner; she helped me come out swinging, optimistic for the win.

And the adventure continues...

# 14: DIVORCE



I made it through the discovery process and diagnosis of CF. So, where do I go from here? Typically one would get support from one's spouse, family, and friends. In my case, two out of three wasn't bad. I received tremendous support from my brother and unwavering support from friends near and far. The only response I received from the siren was, "I want a divorce. I did not sign-up to be a caregiver."

Before I continue, I need to give a brief history lesson regarding the Jewish culture, as it pertains to a wedding ceremony. The first part of the wedding is the signing of the Ketubah. The second part of the wedding is the ceremony itself.

In this ceremony, there is a part called the seven blessings. These aspects of the ceremony go back to days of shepherds and simple farmers. Modern laws do not recognize the Ketubah or the words and meaning behind them as a contract. Rather, it is more a symbol of the couple's love toward each other and the responsibilities they both have in the marriage. Looking back, it appears the seven blessings were hypocritical in the bride's eyes.

I went through the entire Jewish wedding ceremony, I have a beautiful daughter, and now need to deal with the siren who wants to exit the marriage.

I was completely devastated and angry on so many levels. Why go through the effort of getting married, taking vows, having a child, building a family, to only break it up in less than five years? Why leave knowing that the child's father could die in six months, denying a father time for his daughter to know him and know that her father loved her more than anything in the world? Honestly, to this day, her actions of selfishness and abandonment astonish me.

As the divorce proceeded, a formal parenting plan needed to be completed. It was a legal document that outlined the rights and responsibilities of both parents as it related to the child. It was at this point that I discovered that the siren wanted full custody and have my visitation rights limited to supervised visits only.

She insisted that due to my illness, I was an unfit parent and, therefore, should not be granted any custody. Also, my visits needed to be supervised to avoid psychologically damaging our daughter because "I could die in our daughter's presence." Thus someone should always be present for my safety and hers.

These parenting plan sessions continued over several weeks, and the therapist did not agree with the siren. The final outcome was co-parenting custody with a set scheduled time split between us and no need for supervision. After this agreement was finalized, I thought the hard part was behind me. Only the divorce settlement was left to discuss.

How difficult could that be? Unfortunately, I learned that when someone wants to hurt someone else just for the sheer spite, it can be very difficult.

Just when I thought my health would no longer be an issue in, what myself, family, and friends thought would be simple divorce, the siren brought it up again. This caused me to hire a lawyer who fought for my rights as a father.

My health, which I lived with quietly my entire life, was now put on public display, not because I had the disease my entire life, and not because I beat the odds, but because I could die. Being sick, according to the siren, made me a high-risk parent. Thus, clauses needed to be built into the divorce settlement that would give the siren the freedom to revoke my rights as a parent, provisions that would relinquish any opportunity to see and spend any time with my daughter. Also, she wanted a provision that required me to carry a substantial life insurance policy.

At this point in the process, I was getting tired. I was fighting on both physical and mental fronts, not just with the siren, but with myself. I began to question my resolve. Does being sick prevent me from being the best parent I could be? Fuck No! My mother did it—she had MS all those years and primary custody. She raised two sons who grew up and, in my opinion, turned out well. My illness did not compare to MS. So, no, I would not surrender to the foolish and outlandish claims the siren made. I would stay strong and fight until the fight was done. My daughter would know her father, regardless of the hate and protests coming from the siren.

Close to a year passed. My lawyer, my brother, who was financially helping me, and myself were all getting annoyed with the lack of progress. The opposing legal team wanted statements and depositions from my doctors. Why? They were looking for anything to substantiate their position, including statements in the divorce settlement to revoke my parental rights due to health. Unless the court ordered it, no one could have access to my medical records.

At that point, my lawyer suggested we go to court. The back and forth was getting repetitive. Costs kept increasing, and the siren was under the impression that I was paying her court costs. That misconception was quickly resolved when my lawyer filed a motion with the court for the case to be heard in open court, which meant she became responsible for all legal fees if she lost the case.

One must remember, the question being asked in court is, "Does having CF equate to being a bad or unfit parent? If so, does the other parent have the right to revoke or absolve any parental rights of the other parent?" A court date was set. The clock began to tick. Soon, the entire marriage would be made public record, including any alleged improprieties during the marriage and includes but is not limited to, infidelity, etc.

As the court date grew closer, my attorney received correspondence from the opposing lawyer, saying that they wanted to settle. We declined. They were unwilling to remove all_statements related to my illness from the legal document.

Two days before the court date, they relented. It was not because the siren agreed that illness has nothing to do with being a good or fit parent. Rather, the willingness to settle had to do with money; going to court was going to cost her over $30,000 if she lost.

Morality had nothing do with victory. Wanting to be a present father and parent won out over spite, hate, and greed. The siren wanted to hurt me emotionally and financially. It did not work. She failed. Even today, many years later, she still ignorantly believes that being ill equates to being a bad or unfit parent.

I also have to deal with hearing from my daughter that the siren's alleged long-term boyfriend is referred to as Daddy <fill in boyfriend's name>. How does one cope with hearing that from one's daughter who will always be, "Daddy's little girl?"

I tell myself that one day Sydney will finally recognize what is truth and what is fiction. All children from divorced homes figure it out. The road will always have bumps along the way, yet the destination is still the same, the truth will not be silenced.

My support system was amazing; it still is from my brother to all my friends. All were with me, both emotionally and physically. They offered support not just during the divorce, but as I continue to learn how to live day-by-day with CF. I never gave up; I never surrendered.

And the adventure continues...

# 15: THE GREATEST GIFT

The truth is that all great men have had great mothers. Great women have had, as a rule, great fathers.
–Robert Green Ingersoll

Entering marriage and becoming a father is the most rewarding life experience one can ever hope to achieve.

However, having a child with the siren proved difficult. We tried conceiving a child via the traditional method; it didn't work. We tried alternative methods, ranging from acupuncture, herbs, organic eating, yoga—if it was on the Internet, we tried it. Nothing. The siren was getting frustrated; so was I. We decided to consult a specialist.

The first step was an exam for the siren and a plastic cup for me. My test results came back okay. I had swimmers! However, the doctor found large cysts and scarring inside the siren. The doctor asked the siren if she had any past uterine medical procedures, and she answered yes. I was taken off-guard and surprised. She never shared this with me before or after we were married. Also, I didn't know that these procedures could prevent a woman from having children.

What else was she hiding from the doctor or me? As the exam continued, signposts kept popping up, and I kept ignoring them. Our only remaining option was to attempt in vitro fertilization (IVF). However, before IVF could be attempted, the siren needed surgery to remove baseball-size uterine cysts. If the procedure caused internal damage, nothing could be done to change that fact. We just had to hope and pray that any damage was not significant enough to prevent the siren from bearing children.

IVF is one of the more widely known types of assisted reproductive technology (ART), and it works by using a combination of medicines and surgical procedures to help sperm fertilize an egg. These medicines and procedures help the fertilized egg implant in the woman's uterus.

The first step is for the woman to take medication that makes several of her eggs mature and ready for fertilization. Then the doctor takes the eggs out of the woman's body and mixes them with sperm in a lab; this helps the sperm fertilize as many eggs as possible. Then, the doctor puts one or more fertilized eggs, embryos at this point, directly into the woman's uterus. Pregnancy occurs if any of the embryos implants in the uterine lining.

IVF has many steps, and it takes several months to complete the whole process. Sometimes it works on the first try, but many people need more than one round of IVF to get pregnant. IVF increases your chances of pregnancy if you are having fertility problems, but results are not guaranteed. Everyone's body is different, and IVF does not work for everyone.

We went through two rounds of IVF, which proved to be an emotional and trying time for both of us.

The feeling of lack of control over the situation and the desired outcome was beyond words. Also, I continued to wonder if the siren had kept anything else to herself, which could affect the desired result? I'll never know.

Egg-harvest day arrived. At this point, the process is literally in the hands of the doctors, and to my delight, we eventually had six viable embryos. My dream of having a family was coming true. I was happy.

An embryo was implanted in the siren's uterus. The damage caused by the cysts and the procedures did not prevent full-term pregnancy. Our miracle child was brought into this world nine long months later. I cried and thanked God for bringing happiness into my life.

This chapter of my life was composed of both an unbelievable joy and a sadness that will follow me for the rest of my days. When the siren became pregnant, I did not know I had CF. The brightest part of this chapter was the birth of Sydney and becoming a father. I will say it again, "Thank you, God."

The darkest part of this chapter is the story of what happened to the remaining embryos. I wanted Sydney to have a brother or sister. The words of my mother and father rang in my head, "When we are gone, you and your brother will only have each other. You are each other's family, never forget that." As the old saying goes, "It takes two to tango."

The siren did not want to bring another life into this world and not be able to give them everything. "It's better to have one and be able to provide comfort than to struggle with two."

Even now, in my heart and mind, I feel this was, without a doubt, the wrong decision. But, yet again, money was the siren's only motivation—money over the family, money over a brother or sister. No underlying medical reason existed to prevent giving Sydney a sibling. Rather, it was the myopic vision of life quality and perception of possible monetary issues that prevented a second child. People find a way; the keyword is people.

My bro and I are both parents of only children. Both of us have daughters, and our daughters are close to each other, as well as their fathers. Both look alike and act alike.

The remaining embryos were destroyed. Now, and I imagine into the future, when my daughter asks why she does not have a brother or sister, I shed a tear of sadness and regret.

The experience of creating a child and the lack of interest in creating a sibling was a glaring signpost.

I should have seen the signs—the lying or withholding information about a previous medical procedure, the lack of emotions in signing the destruction document for the remaining embryos.

As I write this, I look at my daughter, and I wish I could go back in time to tell Sydney's mom that money is not the world. The world needs families. Yet, conveying these thoughts would have fallen on deaf ears.

God was talking, was I not listening? Was I mourning? To close out this dark chapter, all I can say, as a parent, I will cherish Sydney to the end-of-my-days. When it comes time to stand in front of God, I will admit my mistakes. Will the siren?

And the adventure continues...

# 16: AN OPEN LETTER TO SYDNEY

I have thought a lot about my daughter and what life lies ahead of her. I hope to be with her for many milestones. However, as my doctors have told me, the disease always wins. So, with that bit of knowledge, I want her to know what her daddy would say to her about the road that lies ahead of her.

## A LETTER TO MY SYD

One day you will ask me, "Daddy, what was it like when you were dating?" I will then freeze like a deer caught in the headlights.

"How should I answer a question like that?" I'll wonder. Especially for a young girl, curious about what she's observed in school. Should I exercise my Fifth Amendment Constitutional rights? No, I do not want to be that overprotective parent; I want you to listen to my thoughts.

I do not know what the future of dating will look like for you many years from now or how men will treat you. And I know now, as much as I'd like to, I cannot protect you from all the land-mines and jackals running rampant. You will have to learn to face them on your own.

But I can tell you what to look for. *Look for honor.* Look for integrity, selflessness, sacrifice, and compassion. Find those who champion justice and fidelity. But above all, seek men who emulate humility and meekness. Do not, as so many others do, be deceived into thinking these traits are a weakness. *Meekness is strength wrapped in humility, my dear daughter. It is a strength under control in a world where so many are out of control.*

Do not confuse velvet words and simply holding a door open as honor. Instead, observe how he treats others, your waiter, the homeless, and the marginalized. If you see how he treats those at their highs and lows, you'll know how he will treat you during your high and low points. Heed this wisdom and do not become disillusioned, for honorable men will still break your heart.

A dishonorable man will break up with you via text, Snapchat—if that still exists—or simply ignore you, called ghosting in today's language. But an honorable man will break your heart face-to-face.

Do not despair, my daughter, for as you read this, you may be tempted to believe that honorable men disappeared in the years before you were born. No, they still exist. However, you must search to find them, and that may take many years. It took me years to find your mom. To this day, I know I found a diamond in the "mine of life."

In your search, though, you will encounter many men without honor. Do not blame them, for their fathers did not know how to teach their sons to walk like a man. Many grew up without a male figure to explain what honor and integrity look like. Feel compassion for them instead. Point them to other men you see acting in honorable ways.

I leave you with this in closing, Syd. When you were born, my heart was yours, and I wanted nothing more than to protect you, kiss your face, tickle your tummy, and watch you smile.

One day, I hope to meet the man who feels the same way. However, I do not need to know or want to know about the tickling of the tummy!

All my love,
Daddy (DaDa)

# 17: LULLABY

Every night, before or after Sydney falls asleep, I sing this lullaby to her. She might not hear me, or she might think, "I get it, Daddy, you love me!"

"Yes, yes, I do, my darling daughter. I love you, 3000!"

## Lullaby

Goodnight, goodnight
It's time now to sleep
The moon's watching over
You and your dreams
Goodnight, goodnight
My sweet little one
Tomorrow your eyes
They will light up the sun

But goodnight, goodnight
Sweet dreams for now
Drift off to sleep
On your pillow of clouds
Goodnight, goodnight
My sweet little friend
Tomorrow's adventures
They will soon begin
Tomorrow's adventures
Will soon begin

# 18: EPILOGUE

A true epilogue is removed from the story in time or space. That's the reason it is called an 'Epilogue'; the label serves to alert the reader that the story itself is over, but we are going to now see a distant result or consequence of that story.
–Nancy Kress

I am on my own now. I am over the divorce. I enrolled in online learning at the Sloan School of Business (MIT), and most importantly, I am a single dad who is present for my daughter.

Sydney and I have gone on several Daddy/Daughter vacations. In 2018, not even a year after the divorce—remember how the siren wanted to limit my visits to only supervisory—we went for a week-long vacation to Disneyland in California, just the two of us.

A father who has lived with CF his whole life took his daughter across the country for a solo trip to the happiest place on earth! No oxygen. No caregivers. No interference from the siren. Just pure, uninterrupted Daddy/Daughter fun.

In 2019 we went back to California. The theme of this adventure was "visiting friends who are family."

For a whole week, every day was different. We even had the misfortune of experiencing two earthquakes.

Each year we have a Daddy/Daughter photoshoot. Many of the photos adorn our yearly holiday card, along with vacation photos. More importantly, it gives Sydney sequential memories with her dad. Every time I take her to or pick her up from school, I take photos. Why? Over time, she will have a chronological digital photo album of every time she was with her dad. I keep what Hawkeye, the doctor, always said in the back of my mind, "The disease always wins." Maybe? But not today. I am giving my daughter as many positive memories as I can. I will do so until the house calls.

We fly drones! We camp in our basement with sleeping bags inside a fully-built tent. We feed ducks by the lake, play board games, and have other numerous awesome Daddy/Daughter moments. All captured digitally and in her memories.

Finally, I am working towards getting back into the workforce. Just because I have now been labeled disabled by society does not mean I have to accept it.

I get stronger every day, though I might not run marathons or win a strong-man competition. Are those accomplishments any more important or significant than being a present and an engaged father first and foremost? In my mind, those are accomplishments for one's ego, not for a daughter, who needs her father more than he needs another medal or ribbon on a corkboard. What is more important for her future? I will do anything and everything physically possible to ensure she has one.

Just because one person abandoned me in life does not make me any less loving or caring as a father or as a partner. Yes, I would like to find a partner to share life with. For now, I am putting a pin in that. Because now, my life is about my daughter.

When I know she is ready for that thing called life, I can smile and realize I did the best I could with what I had. And who knows, maybe somewhere along this continuing journey, I just might bump into someone who wants to join me, but until then...the adventure continues...

# 19: ACKNOWLEDGEMENTS

I believe individuals are brought into one's life at a time when they are needed. All these people were brought into my life during my journey. Although we do not talk every day, they continue to be a source of enlightenment, encouragement, deep friendship, and support. They might not know it, but they will now.

Alex Autry
Angela Maske
Anna Hutcheson
Brian Shield
Carol Pierannunzi
Frani Green
Fred Bronson
Jennifer Pope
Jill Brevda
John Hutcheson, III
Joy DiBenedetto
Kay Zussman
Khaki Jones
Laura Dees
Leslie Johnson
Mary Davis, LMTE
McCartney Cox

Steve Broadway, LPTA
Steven Fortt
Todd Daniel
Wendy Edwards
Yvonne Garner

**And of course, my family (you know who you are!)**

# 20: KEEP IN TOUCH

Make it a habit to tell people thank you. To express your appreciation, sincerely and without the expectation of anything in return. Truly appreciate those around you, and you'll soon find many others around you. Truly appreciate life, and you'll find that you have more of it.

–Ralph Marston

I want to thank everyone who purchased this book, and those who went along on this journey with me. I sincerely appreciate all of you!

Also, I would like you to know if you are going through a medical journey with CF or something else, always remember you are not alone.

As I was on my journey, I found solace in writing. I started a blog many years ago, www.blindsidedbycf.com. Feel free to visit it.

If you have a story to tell, want to share your ups and downs of your journey, or you want someone to talk to about your CF journey, reach out and contact me through the website. I would love to hear from you.

No one should feel alone or helpless as they navigate the complexities of the healthcare system. No one should feel alone or helpless as they travel on their journey. There are resources for CF patients. Some are:

Cystic Fibrosis Foundation:
https://www.cff.org/

Healthwellfoundation:
https://www.healthwellfoundation.org/

The above foundations are wonderful resources for anyone with CF. May your journey be safe. I will say it again, just as a reminder, you are never alone.

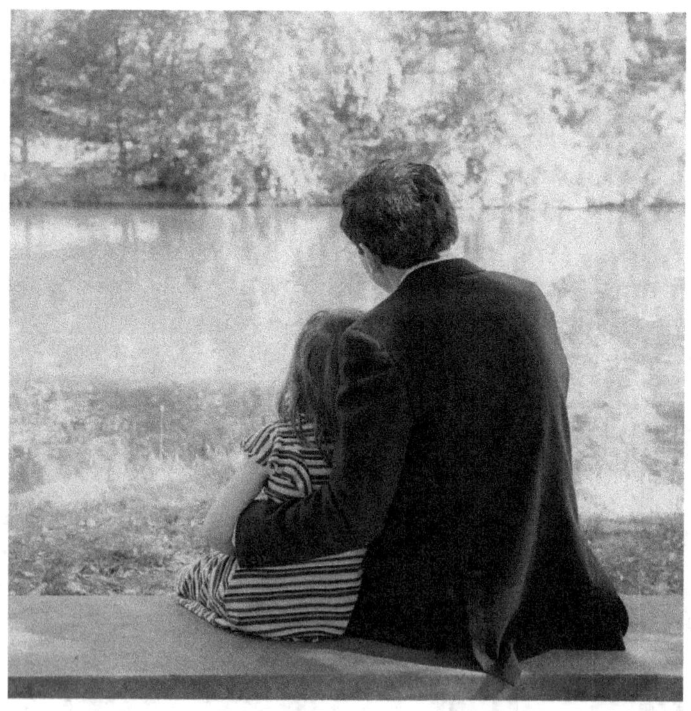

# DISCLAIMER

I would like to thank everyone who has read my drafts, reviewed my artwork, and had to listen to me till the early morning hours.

I have been corrected on minor points, mostly chronology. Someone claims a person who I describe as beautiful was actually quite ugly. I've allowed these points to stand because this is a book of memory, and memory has its own story to tell. Many of the accounts and actions were documented in my journals. I have done my best to make it an accurate account.

Some names and identifying details have been changed to protect the privacy of individuals.

This book is not intended as a substitute for the medical advice of physicians. The reader should regularly consult a physician in matters relating to his/her health and particularly with respect to any symptoms that may require diagnosis or medical attention.